DEVELOPMENTAL NEUROPSYCHOL
Copyright © 2004, Lawrence Erlbaum As:

New Perspectives on Cognitive and Behavioral Outcome After Childhood Closed Head Injury

Maureen Dennis
Department of Psychology
Hospital for Sick Children
Toronto, Ontario, Canada

Harvey S. Levin
Cognitive Neuroscience Laboratory
Departments of Physical Medicine and Rehabilitation,
Neurosurgery, and Psychiatry and Behavioral Sciences
Baylor College of Medicine
Houston, TX

Childhood closed head injury differs from adult head injury in some significant aspects. In this special issue, we attempt to provide an overview of current approaches to the study of childhood closed head injury. We will explore some issues particularly pertinent to children, such as age at head injury and time since head injury, within a context of new developments in the cognitive decomposition of language, memory, and executive function; new perspectives on the interface of cognitive and neuropsychiatric function; and recent advances in neuroimaging in pediatric populations.

Unlike adult head injury, childhood head injury occurs against a background of ongoing physical and cognitive development. One consequence of this is that age and time variables may be significant moderators of the effects of a closed head injury sustained during childhood. The same variable that moderates cognitive effects throughout the life span, such as time since injury, may exert its effects differently in adults and children.

Requests for reprints should be sent to Maureen Dennis, Department of Psychology, Hospital for Sick Children, 555 University Ave., Toronto, Ontario, Canada M5G 1X8. E-mail: maureen.dennis@sickkids.ca

Behavioral changes over time represent instances of functional plasticity. After an acquired brain insult, such as a closed head injury, cognitive capacities often change with time since injury. This change is an instance of functional plasticity. What occurs throughout the interval between injury and cognitive evaluation is a mix of two factors, one concerned with recovery and the other concerned with development.

Plasticity for recovery is what underlies the restitution and reorganization of functions lost or disrupted by the brain insult; for example, a slowed rate of information processing immediately after the closed head injury may improve to preaccident levels over the course of a year or two. But development is also plastic. With increasing age, new cognitive functions are developed at the same time that other functions are rearranged. Plasticity for development is what supports the young brain in acquiring new functions, skills, and knowledge. After damage to the immature brain, plasticity for recovery co-exists with plasticity for development, and both contribute to long-term cognitive outcome.

Understanding plasticity for development requires also that the developmental point of the injury be specified. Broadly, this concerns age at closed head injury, which is a marker for the developmental processes underlying cognitive change. Age at injury and age at testing correspond to the extent of cortical development and myelination with implications for functional commitment of structures such as prefrontal cortex and its circuitry. An injury disrupting development of a prefrontally guided network may have different implications for cognitive function relative to a similar injury in an adult who has well-developed systems for working memory and other prefrontally mediated networks. Cognitive skills emerging at the time of injury might also be especially vulnerable to the effects of severe injury, possibly due to disruption of functional commitment of relevant brain regions and diminished opportunities for learning associated with hospitalization and rehabilitation.

It is timely to revisit the issues of age at injury and time since injury. It is especially timely to review abilities such as working memory as a function of age at injury, and to consider academic skills, so tied to age-based instruction, in relation to age variables. Equally timely is the new focus on longitudinal studies of children after closed head injury with appropriate control groups, which can elucidate issues of recovery and development.

In revisiting these issues, it is possible to capitalize on new advances in neuropsychological measures. In an earlier research era, childhood closed head injury was studied with reference to adult norms and expectations. In a subsequent research era, it was recognized that standard psychometric tests might not evaluate developmentally appropriate functions for children after closed head injury, and the interest shifted to establishing measures of developmentally important skills, such as those involved in executive functions and metacognition. The available of more developmentally appropriate outcome measures has advanced the study of cognitive outcomes in childhood head injury.

Outcome itself has come to be more broadly defined. The concept of outcome has been expanded to include a range of neuropsychological and neuropsychiatric outcomes, which are proving to bear a complex relation to cognitive function. The broader assessment of behavior and neuropsychiatric function has greatly enriched our understanding of the consequences of childhood closed head injury.

Finally, advances in neuroimaging in childhood conditions, such as closed head injury, have advanced knowledge in at least three ways. It has allowed the delineation of injury severity in terms of actual effects on the brain, facilitated the study of brain structure–functional outcome relations, and provided an opportunity to investigate reorganization of function.

DEVELOPMENTAL NEUROPSYCHOLOGY, 25(1&2), 5–20
Copyright © 2004, Lawrence Erlbaum Associates, Inc.

Prospective Memory in Pediatric Traumatic Brain Injury: A Preliminary Study

Stephen R. McCauley
Cognitive Neuroscience Laboratory
Department of Physical Medicine and Rehabilitation
Baylor College of Medicine
Houston, TX

Harvey S. Levin
Cognitive Neuroscience Laboratory
Departments of Physical Medicine and Rehabilitation,
Neurosurgery, and Psychiatry and Behavioral Sciences
Baylor College of Medicine
Houston, TX

Prospective memory (PM) performance was investigated in a preliminary study of children and adolescents ages 10–19 in 3 groups: individuals with orthopedic injuries (not involving the head) requiring hospitalization (Ortho, $N = 15$), mild traumatic brain injury (TBI, $N = 17$), and severe TBI ($N = 15$). All participants with TBI were at least 5 years postinjury and participants in the Ortho group were at least 3 years postinjury. The PM task involved reporting words presented in blue during a category decision task in which words were presented in several different colors and participants were to determine which of two categories the word belonged. Participants were asked to make their choices as quickly as possible. After a 10- to 15-min intervening computer task in which all words were presented in black letters, a large proportion of participants with mild or severe TBI failed to indicate any blue words when they appeared. After a reminder to perform the PM task was given to all at the same point in the task, PM performance increased in the Ortho and Mild TBI groups, but remained comparably impaired in the Severe TBI group. Reaction time (RT) data

Requests for reprints should be sent to Stephen R. McCauley, Cognitive Neuroscience Laboratory, Department of Physical Medicine and Rehabilitation, Baylor College of Medicine, 6560 Fannin Street, Ste. 1144, Houston, TX 77030. E-mail: mccauley@bcm.tmc.edu indicated that mean RT was slower with increasing TBI severity. Further, there was a significant cost in RT for performing the PM task during the ongoing category decision task for all groups. The cost in terms of slowed RT increased with greater TBI severity.

Prospective memory (PM) differs from other forms of memory in that PM is the recall of intentions to be performed in the future instead of events or information recalled from the past (collectively referred to as retrospective memory [RM]). Several types of PM have been theoretically defined on the basis of the specific characteristics of the retrieval context, including event-based (E-B), time-based (T-B), and activity-based (A-B) PM. Event-based PM involves the presence of an external cue (e.g., when a timer goes off, or when you see a colleague) to prompt the performance of an intention (e.g., take the cake out of the oven, or give the colleague a message). Time-based PM tasks are intentions to be carried out at a certain time (e.g., an appointment at 3 o'clock today) or within a given time frame (phone a colleague in 30 min). Activity-based PM involves the performance of an intention when there is a break between tasks and the timing of performance is self-determined (e.g., take a pill either before or after dinner). Some researchers have postulated that a distinction only needs to be made between E-B and T-B PM tasks (Einstein & McDaniel, 1990) or between appointment-keeping intentions (T-B) or performing an intention before or after another (A-B), as Harris does (Harris, 1984). Kvavilashvili (Kvavilashvili, 1990, as cited in Kvavilashvili & Ellis, 1996) has suggested that A-B intentions are distinct from E-B and T-B in that the A-B intentions do not require the interruption of ongoing activities.

PM IN NORMALLY DEVELOPING CHILDREN

PM research has surged in the past 10 to 20 years, particularly due to advances in laboratory methods in normal aging (Einstein, Holland, McDaniel, & Guynn, 1992; Einstein & McDaniel, 1990; McDaniel & Einstein, 1993). Although much light has been shed on the components affecting PM performance in research of the young adults and the elderly, surprisingly little research has been carried out in children and adolescents. In contrast to the extensive literature detailing memory development in normal children and memory deficits in children and adolescents with traumatic brain injury (TBI), scant work has been done with PM in children and adolescents either with or without cerebral compromise. It appears that PM begins developing early in life as PM ability has been reported in children as young as 2 to 4 years (Sommerville, Wellman, & Cultice, 1983). In this study, 2- to 4-year-olds were instructed to remind their mothers to perform certain actions (i.e., reminding their mothers to get ice cream) anywhere from 5 min to 8 hr in the future. Up to 80% of the children successfully performed the future intention. Winograd (Winograd, 1988) speculated that PM might be expected to manifest itself early in development because remembering to carry out an intention may result in reward. Many early studies of PM in young children have focused on specific aspects of an external retrieval cue (Kreutzer, Leonard, & Flavell, 1975; Meacham & Colombo, 1980; Wellman, Ritter, & Flavell, 1975) and its effect on performance. These studies demonstrated that children tend to rely on external cues (e.g., placing to-be-remembered object in obvious locations, leaving a note to oneself, etc.) to aid and sometimes improve PM performance. However, this finding has not been universal (Meacham & Dumitru, 1976). Children 4 to 9 years of age understand that a retrieval cue should be associated with a target intention, but they have difficulty in choosing efficient retrieval cues (specific and informative vs. ambiguous), which leads to misinterpretation of the cues (Beal, 1985). Guajardo and Best (2000) reported that incentives and external cues did not consistently improve performance.

Variables other than external cue have been the focus of study. For instance, greater intervening or ongoing task complexity was found to negatively impact performance of a novel PM task compared to a habitual (frequently performed) PM task in high school students (Wichman & Oyasato, 1983). Kvavilashvili and her colleagues (Kvavilashvili, Messer, & Ebdon, 2001) reported that PM performance was better in a no-interruption condition compared to interruption, suggesting how sensitive PM can be to interference in young children. Time monitoring is another important factor in successful T-B PM tasks. Ceci and Bronfenbrenner (1985) found that 10- and 14-year-olds used similar time-monitoring strategies, but the frequency of time monitoring (clock watching) differed depending on context; there was a U-shaped function of clock watching (very frequent initially and again shortly before the target time approached) in the home setting, but a steadily increasing linear function in the laboratory setting. Passolunghi and her colleagues (Passolunghi, Brandimonte, & Cornoldi, 1995) found that 10-year-olds benefited from visual encoding of the E-B PM cue versus practicing by pressing a key in conjunction with the event cue. Surprisingly, 14-year-olds demonstrated the reverse effect of these encoding manipulations. In contrast to adult memory research, child PM studies (Ceci et al., 1985; Guajardo & Best, 2000; Kreutzer et al., 1975; Kvavilashvili et al., 2001; Meacham et al., 1980; Passolunghi et al., 1995; Schwanenflugel, Fabricius, & Alexander, 1994; Sommerville et al., 1983) have involved a wide range of retention intervals and specific variables on very different tasks related to PM. As a result, there is currently no clear pattern of development of PM abilities emerging from the existing literature.

Little research has been conducted investigating and describing a developmental model of PM. As an initial step in this direction, Schwanenflugel and her colleagues (Schwanenflugel et al., 1994) found that 8-year-olds conceptualize memory as a global construct whereas 10-year-olds are able to distinguish internal and external retrieval cues as well as discern that PM is different from free recall in that

PM requires a planning component for successful performance. Recently, Kerns (2000) has used a computer game-like task to study development of PM abilities in children ages 6–12 years. Her results revealed a robust age effect, and PM performance on this task was correlated with several measures of executive function, even after controlling for age effects. This work is a significant move forward as researchers work to uncover the mechanisms that are involved in normal PM functioning in children and at what rate it evolves.

PM IN CHILDREN WITH TBI

To date, there have been very few studies of PM deficits in children with either acquired or developmental brain dysfunction. Of those, one is a case study of rehabilitating PM deficits in an adolescent with spina bifida using an on-board computer mounted to his wheelchair (Flannery, Butterbaugh, Rice, & Rice, 1997) and two others include children and adolescents with severe TBI (McCauley & Levin, 2000, 2001). This lack of study is surprising as the estimated incidence of acquired brain injury in children in the United States ranges from 180/100,000 (Kraus, 1995) to 200–300/100,000 (Jagger, Levine, Jane, et al., 1984). These injuries are major contributors to developmental disability (Brown, Chadwick, Shaffer, Rutter, & Traub, 1981; Michaud, Duhaime, & Batshaw, 1993; Rutter, 1998). Approximately 17,000 children in the United States are disabled by a TBI annually (Kraus, 1995; Kraus, Fife, & Conroy, 1987; Kraus, Rock, & Hemyari, 1990). A considerable body of work has been amassed in RM deficits in children with TBI (Hannay & Levin, 1979; Hannay & Levin, 1989; Hanten et al., 2000; Levin & Eisenberg, 1979; Levin, Eisenberg, Wigg, & Kobayashi, 1982; Levin & Goldstein, 1986; Levin et al., 1994; Levin, Fletcher, Kusnerik, & Kufera, 1996; Novack, Kofoed, & Crosson, 1995). The lack of investigation into PM following TBI is surprising because it has serious implications for the day-to-day aspects of adaptive behavior of children and adolescents. For instance, typical examples of PM failures may include failing to (a) take routine medications (on their own or with the supervision of the school nurse), (b) complete errands, (c) show up for appointments in school or during free time, (d) bring home special permission slips to be signed, (e) follow instructions at school to be performed independently later in the school day, (f) call their parents at work when they return home from school, (g) return books to the library, (h) complete homework assignments or even failing to take completed homework back to school. Clearly the effects of PM failures are likely demonstrated beyond school, and the current literature on sequelae of pediatric TBI does not address the nature of these deficits in children and adolescents.

What is currently known about PM performance in children with severe TBI comes from preliminary studies employing tasks that appear to be ecologically valid within the context of a neuropsychological assessment or cognitive psychology laboratory procedure conducted by McCauley and Levin (2000, 2001). In these studies, children (6–16 years of age at testing) who were at least 2 years postinjury with a severe TBI were significantly impaired at recalling E-B and A-B PM tasks compared to a similar-aged group of normally developing children. There was a trend for greater impairment as the number of intentions increased from one (immediately placing their hands in their lap after a bell went off) to two (picking up a red pencil and saying "I'm ready" after a verbal cue from the examiner) in E-B and A-B tasks. Given the small sample size, it is difficult to interpret the robustness of the age effect for these tasks given that an age effect was found in the E-B tasks, but was absent in the A-B tasks.

Injury effects are frequently reported in pediatric TBI studies of declarative memory. It is plausible to assume that similar injury severity effects will manifest in studies of pediatric PM resulting in greater impairment with increasing severity. What remains unclear is if children with a mild TBI will demonstrate an appreciable deficit in PM functioning.

METHOD

Participants

All children participating in this study spoke English fluently. Informed consent was obtained from all individuals with an experimental protocol approved by the Baylor College of Medicine Institutional Review Board. Children were recruited as part of a larger, long-term follow-up study of children and young adults who were at least 5 years post-TBI who had been prospectively recruited (Parkland Hospital and Children's Medical Center in Dallas, Texas; Hermann Hospital, Ben Taub General Hospital, and Texas Children's Hospital in Houston, Texas) for previous studies conducted through our laboratory or (primarily for children with orthopedic injuries children) who were recruited through advertisements at local YMCA summer camp and other public facilities in the community. TBI severity was determined through the lowest postresuscitation Glasgow Coma Scale (GCS) score (Teasdale & Jennett, 1974). This sample includes children and adolescents ranging in age from 10 to 19 years: 15 children with severe TBI (postresuscitation GCS ≤ 8), 17 children with mild TBI (postresuscitation GCS 13–15 with or without trauma-related abnormalities on hospital admission head CT), and 15 children who had sustained orthopedic injuries (i.e., broken bones) not involving the head (Ortho) at least 3 years prior to their participation in this study. Children recruited for the Ortho group were excluded if they had a history of major psychiatric disorder, pervasive developmental delay, learning or attention disorder, or prior head injury. The mean ages of the groups were 15.73 ($SD = 1.94$, range 12–19 years) for the Severe TBI group, 15.29 (SD = 2.08, range 10–19 years) for the Mild TBI group, and 15.13 (SD = 2.45, range 11–19 years) for the Ortho group. The groups did not differ significantly by age, $F(2, 44) = .31$, $p = .73$. Groups did not differ by gender composition, $\chi^2(2, N = 46) = 2.14$, $p = .34$, or socioeconomic status (as measured by mean parental education level, $p > .05$).

Materials

All computer testing was performed using Macintosh Powerbook and Psyscope software (Cohen, MacWhinney, Flatt, & Provost, 1993) for stimulus presentation and data recording. The word list for the category decision tasks was derived from category exemplars with low age of acquisition from the Oxford Psycholinguistic Database. Words in each block were balanced for age of acquisition.

Procedure

Before starting a series of computer tasks, participants were told that during the course of the tasks they would see words presented in different colors. When they saw a word presented in blue letters, they were to tell the examiner immediately that they had seen a blue word. Following these instructions, participants engaged in a separate, verbal-based computer task (this task was to investigate issues not related to this paper and essentially served as a complex filler task) for 10 to 15 min during which time all words appeared in black letters. The participants then began a category decision task in which they were to decide which of two categories a word belonged (e.g., fruits and furniture) by pressing either "N" or "C" on the keyboard depending on the categories assigned to these keys as quickly as possible. Words presented on the screen remained visible until the participant made a category decision, which was followed by a blank screen for 500 msec before the next word appeared. The category decision task comprised 8 blocks (8 pairs of categories) of 20 trials each. The first four trials of each block were intended as practice and not included in the reaction time (RT) data. Participants were given no warning that this task would include blue words. Three blue words occurred in the first three blocks. Independent of the participant's performance, a reminder was given at the start of the fourth block that the participant should tell the examiner any time a word was presented in blue letters. No blue words appeared during the fourth block, but two blue words appeared during the course of blocks five and six. At the start of block seven, participants were told that there would be no more blue words to watch for. For analysis, RTs for blocks one through three were combined to form Block 1 (ongoing task with PM task), blocks four through six were summed to form Block 2 (ongoing task with reminder of PM task), and blocks seven and eight were summed to form Block 3 (ongoing task without PM task). Dependent measures included the RTs for each trial (excluding practice trials and trials on which blue words were presented), and the number of reports of blue words before and after a cue reminder. The blue words and their positions were the same for all participants. The examiner was positioned near the participant so that the words on the computer screen were visible, allowing the examiner to record correct recall of the blue word (PM behavioral data) or any false alarms that may have occurred.

Analyses

The level of significance was set at $\alpha = .05$ unless otherwise noted. Given the preliminary exploratory nature of this experiment, alpha levels for post hoc analyses remained at .05; this has the effect of increasing the probability of committing a Type-I error, but this procedure was considered more acceptable than committing a Type-II error and missing future potential avenues of study. When performing chi-square analyses, Fisher's Exact Test was used when proportions were more extreme than 80–20 or when cell membership for any given cell was ≤5. RT data was analyzed for the presence and elimination of outliers using Cook's D procedure. Due to the L-shaped distribution, RTs were converted to a logarithmic scale, but this failed to produce a normal distribution. The RTs were then inverted (i.e., $1/X$), which satisfactorily approximated a normal distribution. Subsequent analyses on RTs were conducted with the inverted RT data. RTs for practice trials and trials during which a blue word (PM cue) was presented were not included in the analyses.

RESULTS

Behavioral Data

Due to examiner error, behavioral data was unavailable for 3 participants, one in each group. The number of blue words identified in Block 1 (the actual start of the blue word task without reminder) was analyzed using the Kruskal-Wallis procedure for nonparametric one-way analysis of variance (ANOVA), which indicated significant between-group differences ($p = .0003$). In post hoc analyses using the Mann-Whitney U test, the Mild TBI ($Z = 2.76, p < .005$) and Severe TBI groups ($Z = 3.60, p = .0006$) performed significantly poorer compared to the Ortho group. Although the Severe TBI group performed more poorly than the Mild TBI group, this difference failed to reach significance ($Z = -1.38, p = .09$). Data from Block 1 were then collapsed to determine the proportion of each of the three groups who spontaneously indicated the presence of at least one of the three blue words (which was considered sufficient evidence that the participant had remembered to perform the intention) versus those who failed to indicate any blue words. Although only 10 to 15 min elapsed between the PM instructions and the start of the PM task, the proportion of spontaneous PM performance differed dramatically (Ortho 71.4%,

Mild 25%, Severe 7.1%), and this result was quite significant (Fisher's Exact Test, $p = .001$). Post hoc analyses indicated that the Ortho group differed significantly from the Mild TBI (Fisher's Exact Test, $p < .02$) and Severe TBI groups (Fisher's Exact Test, $p < .0007$); the Mild and Severe TBI groups did not differ significantly (Fisher's Exact Test, $p = .21$).

In a similar manner to that of data from Block 1, the number of blue words participants reported in Block 2 (PM performance following reminder) was analyzed through the Kruskal-Wallis procedure, which failed to find overall significant group differences ($p = .08$). Follow-up analyses were then conducted to determine if the performance of the Ortho group differed significantly from the Mild or Severe TBI groups. Regarding benefit of a reminder, the Mild TBI group performed at a level comparable to that of the Ortho group ($Z = .42$, $p = .34$), but the Severe TBI group did not appear to benefit from the reminder ($Z = 2.08$, $p < .03$) compared to the Ortho group. Although the Mild TBI group recalled more words following the reminder compared to the Severe TBI group, the difference failed to reach significance ($Z = -1.52$, $p = .07$). Given the large proportion of participants with TBI who failed to indicate blue words in Block 1, analysis turned to the proportions of subjects who indicated at least one of the two blue words presented following the PM reminder half-way through the category decision task. Although the groups appeared to differ substantially (Ortho 92.9%, Mild 75.0%, Severe 57.1%), the result was not significant (Fisher's Exact Test, $p = .10$). In follow-up analyses, few in the Severe TBI group appeared to benefit from the reminder to perform the PM task compared to the Ortho group (Fisher's Exact Test, $p < .04$), and the Ortho and Mild TBI groups benefited from the reminder at a comparable rate (Fisher's Exact Test, $p = .21$). Finally, performance of the Mild and Severe TBI groups was examined, revealing that, although a greater proportion of participants in the Mild TBI group appeared to benefit from the reminder of the PM task compared to the Severe TBI group, this difference was not significant (Fisher's Exact Test, $p = .26$).

RT Data

Given that a large proportion of participants in the Severe and Mild TBI groups did not spontaneously perform the PM task (see Figure 1) during Block 1 (thus negating any possible effect of maintaining the intention to perform the PM task in terms of slowed RT), subsequent analyses were performed on Blocks 2 (with PM task) and 3 (without PM task) only. RT data for the full experiment are presented in Figure 2. The inverted RTs (Blocks 2 and 3 combined) were analyzed for main effect of age (faster RTs with increasing age), which was significant, $F(1, 3428) = 8.10$, $p = .004$. Inverted RTs were then analyzed for main effect of group, which was also found to be significant, $F(2, 3427) = 322.71$, $p < .0001$. Post hoc analysis using Tukey adjustment for multiple comparisons (see Figure 3) indicated a significant difference in mean RT between the Ortho and Severe TBI groups ($p < .0001$),

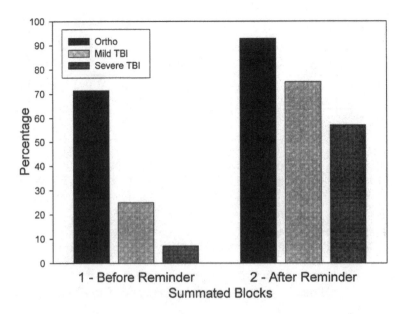

FIGURE 1   Percentage of participants performing the prospective memory task at least once.

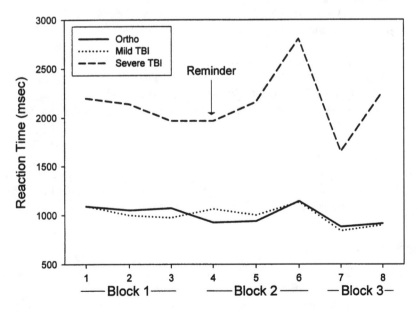

FIGURE 2   Mean reaction times for individual and summated blocks.

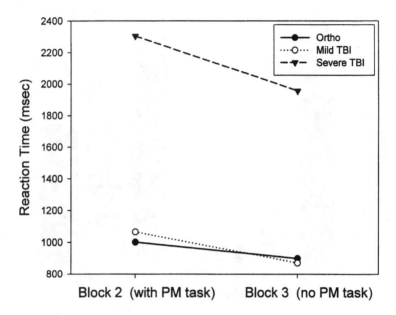

FIGURE 3   Reaction times for summated Blocks 2 and 3.

Ortho and Mild TBI groups ($p = .0006$), and Mild and Severe TBI groups ($p < .0001$). The data was further analyzed using a two-way ANOVA with hierarchical structure such that Block was nested within Group in addition to controlling for the significant age effect. Analysis of Block as a within-subjects factor indicated that the Ortho group RT was significantly faster ($t = -7.58$, $p < .0001$) in Block 3 (no PM task) than Block 2 (PM task), as were the Mild TBI ($t = -8.43$, $p < .0001$) and Severe TBI ($t = -6.52$, $p < .0001$) groups. Using Tukey's procedure for multiple comparisons, groups were then compared for inverted RTs within each block (between-subjects). In Block 2, the Ortho group was significantly faster than those in the Mild TBI group ($p < .02$), who were also faster than the Severe TBI group ($p < .0001$), and those in the Mild TBI group were faster than the Severe TBI group ($p < .0001$). In Block 3, the Ortho and Mild TBI group performed similarly ($p = .35$), but the Ortho was faster than the Severe TBI group ($p < .0001$), and the Mild TBI group was faster than the Severe TBI group ($p < .0001$).

Summary

In summary, these results demonstrated that children and adolescents with chronic mild and severe TBI (at least 5 years) have significant impairments in PM compared to the Ortho comparison group. This was clearly evident when performing a challenging mental task for 10 to 15 min resulted in PM failures for 75.0% and

92.9% of the Mild and Severe TBI participants, respectively. The use of a reminder of the PM task revealed that the Severe TBI group did not benefit from the reminder cue to the degree that the Ortho and Mild TBI groups did; nearly 43% of the Severe TBI participants failed to report a single blue word just moments after being reminded to do so compared to 25% of Mild TBI and only 7.1% of Ortho participants. Regarding the RT data, the Ortho group was quicker than the Mild TBI group, who in turn was quicker than the Severe TBI group within Block 2 and within Block 3, separately. Within-subject analyses revealed that all groups showed a significant cost in terms of RT for performing the PM task with the Severe TBI group demonstrating the greatest cost (see Figure 4).

DISCUSSION

These results are some of the first to describe PM deficits in child and adolescents with mild or severe TBI. Although these data should be viewed with caution given their preliminary and exploratory quality and relatively small sample size, they do present compelling evidence of the chronic nature of PM deficits in pediatric TBI. As all of the TBI participants were at least 5 years postinjury, these deficits can not be argued to be transient and confined to an early postacute recovery period. One

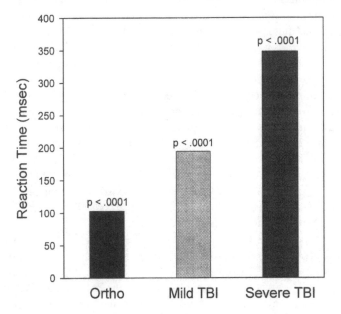

FIGURE 4   Cost in RT for performing PM task (Block 3–Block 2). The significant differences depicted are for within-subjects comparisons.times for summated Blocks 2 and 3.

of the more interesting findings is that the Mild TBI group performed significantly more poorly compared to the Ortho controls not only in terms of RT data, but also on some of the behavioral measures. For instance, following the brief delay between PM instructions and the onset of the task, a large proportion of the Mild TBI participants had forgotten to report the blue words as instructed. This is striking given that the words displayed during the intervening task were presented in black. One might speculate that the sudden appearance of words in different colors would have been a salient cue (or "pop-out" effect) that something different was going on in the category decision task than in the preceding verbal task. The cue for the PM task could hardly have been more closely related than the colored words. In spite of this, many of the Mild TBI and a substantial number of Ortho participants failed to connect this unique cue to the actual PM task. It is interesting to note that both the Ortho and Mild TBI groups benefited from the reminder to perform the PM task as the proportion of participants performing the PM task at least once was not statistically different. Regarding the performance of the Severe TBI group, these children demonstrated substantial improvement in PM after the reminder compared to their performance before (see Figure 1). However, just under half of these participants failed to report a blue word just moments after being reminded to do so, suggesting that a cue can improve PM performance, but clearly it is not fully effective for all children with severe TBI.

An interesting finding was demonstrated in the trend for increasing RTs from block 4 to block 6. This trend was slight, but evident in the Ortho and Mild TBI groups, but was quite pronounced in the Severe TBI group. One possible explanation is that the words were more difficult to categorize in these blocks or that the sequence of the categories was producing an order effect. This appears unlikely as the words were balanced for age of acquisition, which was rather low throughout all blocks. Although speculative, this effect may be due to a build-up of effort (fatigue effect) to maintaining vigilance for the appropriate cue over time to perform the PM task. As there is no RT data of children with TBI performing a PM task for comparison, it is not currently possible to determine the uniqueness of this finding. The Severe TBI group presents another surprising finding in the exaggerated rebound in RT from block 6 to block 7 when released from the PM task, which returns almost as dramatically back to the level demonstrated during blocks 1 and 2. Replication with another sample of children with chronic TBI would help to shed light on these interesting findings.

Performance of the PM task during an ongoing task has a clear and significant effect on RT as demonstrated in the Ortho group (see Figure 4). This "cost" is magnified in the Mild TBI group, in which difference in RT from PM to no PM was twice as great. The great effort required to perform the PM task is evident in the Severe TBI group, in which the cost of PM performance was nearly four times as great as the Ortho group. This level of effort required has serious implications for performance of everyday types of PM tasks. From one moment to the next in daily life, circumstances change that force modification of strategies to recall future intentions. These intentions must be maintained while ongoing attentional and task demands fluctuate. It is easy to see how children with severe TBI would have difficulties in maintaining to-be-performed intentions; recall that only one of the participants in the Severe TBI group remembered to perform the PM task just 10 to 15 min after the instructions were given. Although few lasting deficits are generally found in children sustaining mild TBI, these results suggest that they too are at risk for multiple PM failures in everyday life. Much more study is required to determine what is the extent of PM deficits in children with mild and severe TBI and under what conditions these abilities are most extensively taxed, and what compensatory strategies are most beneficial for these children.

There are some limitations of this study that require acknowledgment. First, the sample size was small, which may have decreased the power for detecting significant differences. However, given the substantial effects demonstrated through Tukey-adjusted level of significance in post hoc analyses of the RT data, this did not appear to be a major concern. However, the small number of targets (blue words) in Blocks 1 and 2 certainly limited the types of analyses that could be performed to nonparametric techniques that are less powerful. Here, too, some effects in planned comparisons were strong enough to emerge leaving post hoc analyses to fall victim to limited power. Future experiments will be designed to allow for parametric analyses of behavioral data to overcome this issue. Second, the RT data from Block 1 was compromised in that a large proportion of participants failed to perform the PM tasks following a relatively brief delay (see Figure 1). What is evident from the figure is that the slowed mean RT of Ortho group in Block 1 resulted from 75% of the participants attending for the E-B PM cue whereas the Mild TBI group appeared equal or superior to the Orthos as only 25% of the group actually was engaged in the PM task. Once the reminder was given, the upward trend in RT is clear in the Mild TBI group as the majority of the group was once again engaged in the PM task. Third, the participants were released from the PM task at the end of the experiment, which could have inflated the difference in RT between the PM versus no-PM conditions; practice effects of performing the decision task could have accrued so that Block 3 was much quicker than if a no-PM condition had preceded the PM condition. Such an effect would be most evident in the Severe TBI group because adults with severe TBI have been shown to have a longer and slower practice effect trajectory in RT measures (Schweinberger, Buse, & Sommer, 1993), which would have resulted in a downward trajectory up to block 4 when the reminder occurred. This also does not necessarily appear to be the case as the Severe TBI group appears to have reached a RT plateau by block 3 and remained stable through block 4 as depicted in Figure 2.

Conclusion

Children with chronic mild or severe TBI demonstrate deficits in PM functioning as measured by behavioral and RT data. Reminding these children of the PM task resulted in significant improvements in PM performance for the Mild TBI group, but not the Severe TBI group. These results have implications for memory deficits in children and adolescents with mild TBI, which have not been demonstrated previously. Further, strategies for improving PM performance in children with chronic severe TBI need to be extended beyond simple task reminders or cues to maximize performance. Motivation may prove to be a useful strategy to manipulate in future studies. Such experiments are currently under development in our laboratory.

ACKNOWLEDGMENTS

This work was supported in part by National Institutes of Health Grant NS–21889, Grant IBIA007 from the International Brain Injury Association (Gerri Hanten, principal investigator), the Clinical Research Centers at Baylor College of Medicine–Texas Children's Hospital, and the University of Texas Health Science Center.

We thank Gerri Hanten for her assistance in designing the prospective memory task. We also thank Rachael Andrews, Ralphanna Barnes, and Allison Franz for their assistance in contacting, recruiting, and testing the participants in this study.

REFERENCES

Beal, C. R. (1985). Development of knowledge about the use of cues to aid prospective retrieval. *Child Development, 56,* 631–642.

Brown, G., Chadwick, O., Shaffer, D., Rutter, M., & Traub, M. (1981). A prospective study of children with head injuries in adulthood III: Psychiatric sequelae. *Psychological Medicine, 11,* 63–78.

Ceci, S. J., & Bronfenbrenner, U. (1985). "Don't forget to take the cupcakes out of the oven": Prospective memory, strategic time-monitoring, and context. *Child Development, 56,* 152–164.

Cohen, J. D., MacWhinney, B., Flatt, M., & Provost, J. (1993). PsyScope: A new graphic interactive environment for designing psychology experiments. *Behavioral Research Methods, Instruments, and Computers, 25,* 257–271.

Einstein, G. O., Holland, L. J., McDaniel, M. A., & Guynn, M. J. (1992). Age-related deficits in prospective memory: The influence of task complexity. *Psychology and Aging, 7,* 471–478.

Einstein, G. O., & McDaniel, M. A. (1990). Normal aging and prospective memory. *Journal of Experimental Psychology: Learning, Memory, and Cognition, 16,* 717–726.

Flannery, M. A., Butterbaugh, G. J., Rice, D. A., & Rice, J. C. (1997). Reminding technology for prospective memory disability: A case study. *Pediatric Rehabilitation, 1,* 239–244.

Guajardo, N. R., & Best, D. L. (2000). Do preschoolers remember what to do? Incentive and external cues in prospective memory. *Cognitive Development, 15,* 75–97.

Hannay, H. J., & Levin, H. S. (1979). *Continuous Recognition Memory Test* [Manual]. Houston, TX: Author.

Hannay, H. J., & Levin, H. S. (1989). Visual continuous recognition memory in normal and closed-head-injured adolescents. *Journal of Clinical & Experimental Neuropsychology, 11,* 444–460.

Hanten, G., Martin, R. C., Hanten, G., Martin, R. C., Hanten, G., & Martin, R. C. (2000). Contributions of phonological and semantic short-term memory to sentence processing: Evidence from two cases of closed head injury in children. *Journal of Memory & Language, 43,* 335–361.

Harris, J. E. (1984). Remembering to do things: A forgotten topic. In J. E. Harris & P. E. Morris (Eds.), *Everyday memory, actions and absent-mindedness* (pp. 71–92). London: Academic.

Jagger, J., Levine, J. I., Jane, J. A., & Rimel, R. W. (1984). Epidemiological features of head injury in predominantly rural population. *Journal of Trauma, 24,* 40–44.

Kerns, K. A. (2000). The CyberCruiser: An investigation of development of prospective memory in children. *Journal of the International Neuropsychological Society, 6,* 62–70.

Kraus, J. F. (1995). Epidemiological features of brain injury in children: Occurrence, children at risk, causes and manner of injury, severity, and outcomes. In S. H. Broman & M. E. Michel (Eds.), *Traumatic head injury in children* (pp. 22–39). New York: Oxford University Press.

Kraus, J. F., Fife, D., & Conroy, C. (1987). Pediatric brain injuries: The nature, clinical course, and deadly outcomes in a defined United States population. *Pediatrics, 79,* 501–507.

Kraus, J. F., Rock, A., & Hemyari, P. (1990). Brain injuries among infants, children, adolescents, and young adults. *American Journal of Diseases of Childhood, 144,* 684–691.

Kreutzer, M. A., Leonard, C., & Flavell, J. H. (1975). Prospective remembering in children. In U. Neisser (Ed.), *Memory observed: Remembering in natural contexts* (pp. 343–348). San Francisco: Freeman.

Kvavilashvili, L. (1990). *Remembering/forgetting intention as a distinct form of memory and the factors that influence it.* Tblisi, Russia: Metsniereba.

Kvavilashvili, L., & Ellis, J. (1996). Varieties of intention: Some distinctions and classifications. In M. A. Brandimonte, G. O. Einstein, & M. A. McDaniel (Eds.), *Prospective memory: Theory and applications* (pp. 23–51). Mahwah, NJ: Lawrence Erlbaum Associates, Inc.

Kvavilashvili, L., Messer, D. J., & Ebdon, P. (2001). Prospective memory in children: The effects of age and task interruption. *Developmental Psychology, 37,* 418–430.

Levin, H. S. (1985). Impairment of remote memory after closed head injury. *Journal of Neurology, Neurosurgery & Psychiatry, 48,* 556–563.

Levin, H. S., Culhane, K. A., Fletcher, J. M., Mendelsohn, D. B., Levin, H. S., Culhane, K. A., et al. (1994). Dissociation between delayed alternation and memory after pediatric head injury: Relationship to MRI findings. *Journal of Child Neurology, 9,* 81–89.

Levin, H. S., & Eisenberg, H. M. (1979a). Neuropsychological impairment after closed head injury in children and adolescents. *Journal of Pediatric Psychology, 4,* 389–402.

Levin, H. S., Eisenberg, H. M., Wigg, N. R., & Kobayashi, K. (1982). Memory and intellectual ability after head injury in children and adolescents. *Neurosurgery, 11,* 668–673.

Levin, H. S., Fletcher, J., Kusnerik, L., & Kufera, J. A. (1996). Semantic memory following pediatric head injury: Relationship to age, severity of injury, and MRI. *Cortex, 32,* 461–478.

Levin, H. S., & Goldstein, F. (1986). Organization of verbal memory after severe closed-head injury. *Journal of Clinical and Experimental Neuropsychology, 8,* 643–656.

McCauley, S. R., & Levin, H. S. (2000). *Prospective memory deficits in children and adolescents sustaining severe closed-head injury.* Presentation at the annual meeting of the Cognitive Neuroscience Society, San Francisco, CA.

McCauley, S. R., & Levin, H. S. (2001). *Prospective memory and executive function in children with severe traumatic brain injury.* Presentation at the 3rd International Conference on Memory (ICOM-3), Valencia, Spain.

McDaniel, M. A., & Einstein, G. O. (1993). The importance of cue familiarity and cue distinctiveness in prospective memory. *Memory, 1,* 23–41.

Meacham, J. A., & Colombo, J. A. (1980). External retrieval cues facilitate prospective remembering in children. *Journal of Educational Research, 73,* 299–301.

Meacham, J. A., & Dumitru, J. (1976). Prospective remembering and external retrieval cues. *Catalog of Selected Documents in Psychology, 6,* 66.

Michaud, L. J., Duhaime, A. C., & Batshaw, M. L. (1993). Traumatic brain injury in children. *Pediatric Clinics of North America, 40,* 553–565.

Novack, T. A., Kofoed, B. A., & Crosson, B. (1995). Sequential performance on the California Verbal Learning Test following traumatic brain injury. *Clinical Neuropsychologist, 9,* 38–43.

Passolunghi, M. C., Brandimonte, M. A., & Cornoldi, C. (1995). Encoding modality and prospective memory in children. *International Journal of Behavioral Development, 18,* 1995–648.

Rutter, M. (1998). Psychological sequelae of brain damage in children. *American Journal of Psychiatry, 138,* 1533–1544.

Schwanenflugel, P. J., Fabricius, W. V., & Alexander, J. (1994). Developing theories of mind: understanding concepts and relations between mental activities. *Child Development, 65,* 1546–1563.

Schweinberger, S. R., Buse, C., & Sommer, W. (1993). Reaction time improvements with practice in brain-damaged patients. *Cortex, 29,* 333–340.

Sommerville, S. C., Wellman, H. M., & Cultice, J. C. (1983). Young children's deliberate reminding. *The Journal of Genetic Psychology, 143,* 87–96.

Teasdale, G., & Jennett, B. (1974). Assessment of coma and impaired consciousness: A practical scale. *Lancet, 2,* 81–84.

Wellman, H. M., Ritter, K., & Flavell, J. H. (1975). Developmental Psychology. *Developmental Psychology, 11,* 780–787.

Wichman, H., & Oyasato, A. (1983). Effects of locus of control and task complexity on prospective remembering. *Human Factors, 25,* 583–591.

Winograd, E. (1988). Some observations on prospective remembering. In M.Gruneberg, P. E. Morris, & R. Sykes (Eds.), *Practical aspects of memory: Current research and issues* (pp. 348–353). New York: Wiley.

DEVELOPMENTAL NEUROPSYCHOLOGY, 25(1&2), 21–36

Working Memory After Mild, Moderate, or Severe Childhood Closed Head Injury

Caroline Roncadin, Sharon Guger, Jennifer Archibald, Marcia
Barnes, and Maureen Dennis

Department of Psychology
Hospital for Sick Children
Toronto, Ontario, Canada

Children with closed head injury (CHI) perform poorly on complex tasks requiring working memory (WM). It is unclear to what extent WM itself is compromised, and whether WM varies with factors related to the CHI, such as injury severity, age at injury, and time since injury. We studied verbal WM in 126 school-age children with CHI, divided into mild, moderate, and severe injury severity groups. WM distributions were significantly skewed toward lower scores in the moderate and severe groups, although the distribution in the mild group was normal. Age at injury and time since injury predicted WM components only for the moderate group. Survivors of moderate or severe childhood CHI have persisting WM deficits limiting the computational workspace required for many cognitive tasks.

Working memory (WM) is a construct referring to the computational ability to relate old information to new, incoming information. WM supports many cognitive processes, from following instructions to understanding written texts and performing mathematical calculations. For this reason, it is considered to be a core cognitive resource.

Current WM models (e.g., Baddeley, 1986; Logie, 1996) emphasize separable components of maintenance (the active retention of information) and manipulation (information processing). Capacity is the amount of information that can be maintained and manipulated in WM at any given time. Increased processing demands, such as the need to simultaneously inhibit irrelevant information, constrain WM

Requests for reprints should be sent to Maureen Dennis, Department of Psychology, Hospital for Sick Children, 555 University Avenue, Toronto, Ontario, Canada M5G 1X8. E-mail: maureen.dennis.sickkids.ca

capacity (Case, 1985; Richardson, 1996; Roncadin, Pascual-Leone, Rich, & Dennis, 2003).

Typically developing children become more efficient with age at maintaining and manipulating information within WM (Cowan, 1997; Hulme & Roodenrys, 1995; Roncadin et al., 2003). Age-related WM improvement is attributed to increased speed of processing (and decreased speed of decay), increased inhibitory control, and the development of knowledge-based (e.g., chunking) and operation-based (e.g., rehearsal) strategies (Barrouillet & Camos, 2001; Bjorklund & Harnishfeger, 1990; Cowan, 1997; Roncadin et al., 2003).

In children, WM efficiency is linked directly to learning and academic competencies, such as reading and arithmetic. Poor WM often coexists with low achievement or specific learning disabilities (Bull & Scerif, 2001; Gathercole & Pickering, 2000; Montgomery, 1995; Passolunghi & Siegel, 2001; Swanson, 1993). In such cases, WM inefficiency is thought to constrain children's ability for cognitive processing and to contribute to their learning difficulties (Hulme & Roodenrys, 1995).

Functional neuroimaging and adult lesion studies dissociate information storage from maintenance and manipulation processes. Storage involves posterior brain regions, whereas maintenance and manipulation are primarily controlled by frontal lobe regions (Awh, Smith, & Jonides, 1995; Fletcher & Henson, 2001; Petrides, 2000; Postle, Berger, & D'Esposito, 1999). WM function may be compromised when the frontal lobes are damaged, as occurs in more than two thirds of severe closed head injury (CHI) cases (Mendelsohn et al., 1992; Yeates, 2000). Moreover, when the CHI is incurred in childhood, during a critical period of rapid frontal lobe maturation, the development of WM may be delayed or arrested (Taylor & Alden, 1997).

Decades of research using a variety of measures of retrospective, declarative memory have established that children with CHI are vulnerable to semantic and episodic memory impairments (Chadwick, Rutter, Shaffer, & Shrout, 1981; Levin, Eisenberg, Wigg, & Kobayashi, 1982; Levin et al., 1996; Roman et al., 1998; Yeates, Blumenstein, Patterson, & Delis, 1995). More recently, WM deficits after childhood CHI have been reported. In the N-back task paradigm, children and adolescents with severe CHI are deficient at visually detecting target letters (Levin et al., 2002) and target words (Proctor, Wilson, Sanchez, & Wesley, 2000). The effects of a primary verbal WM deficit on the development and use of more complex language skills, however, have been inferred in a range of CHI outcome studies. Poor verbal WM after childhood CHI has been associated with sentence comprehension and inferencing difficulties (Barnes & Dennis, 2001; Dennis & Barnes, 1990, 2001; Hanten, Levin, & Song, 1999; Montgomery, 1995; Turkstra & Holland, 1998). Impaired verbal WM also has more widespread consequences in pragmatics and discourse (Barnes & Dennis, 2001; Brookshire, Chapman, Song, & Levin, 2000; Chapman et al., 1992; Dennis & Barnes, 1990, 2000), which, in turn, can affect academic achievement and social adaptation (Ewing-Cobbs et al., this issue).

The effects of CHI on cognitive outcome, including memory, are moderated by injury severity. Consistently, children with severe CHI exhibit poorer memory than those with milder forms of injury. In particular, tests of short- and long-term recall continue to differentiate CHI severity groups several years postinjury (Fay et al., 1994; Levin et al., 1988). The biology of the injury (specifically, the presence of focal damage) can influence the form of memory impairment. In adults, retrospective memory deficits are associated with temporal lobe lesions, whereas frontal lobe damage affects prospective remembering (Palmer & McDonald, 2000).

Cognitive outcome after childhood CHI also varies with developmental status. In comparison to children who sustain their CHI later in development, children injured before age eight typically fail to exhibit expected recovery patterns and exhibit more long-term cognitive impairment (Anderson & Moore, 1995; Verger et al., 2000). A younger age at injury is considered to be a significant risk factor for poor cognitive outcome (Dennis, 1988; Yeates, 2000). Time since injury represents recovery as well as development, and so interacts with the biology and age of the CHI. Recovery in some functional domains can be expected in the immediate postacute period, although new evidence shows that regional and diffuse brain atrophy can occur long after CHI (MacKenzie et al., 2002). As neural maturational processes unfold abnormally, or fail to unfold at all, time since injury can reveal progressive deficits in some, if not all, emerging skills (Dennis, 1988).

In this study, we investigated the maintenance and load aspects of verbal WM in a large sample of children who had sustained a CHI several years earlier. We had five specific aims, concerned respectively with: distributional features of WM performance; the moderating effects of CHI severity, biological, and developmental variables; and, component processes of WM. We aimed to

1. Describe the distribution of WM age percentiles in children with CHI. We hypothesized that the distribution would show a significant positive skew.

2. Examine how CHI severity affects WM. We hypothesized that the distribution of the severe group would show a larger positive skew than in groups with milder injuries, and that WM age percentiles would vary linearly with injury severity, such that they would be below the population mean only in the moderate and severe groups.

3. Evaluate the interaction of severity group and presence of frontal injury in WM age percentiles. We hypothesized that the subgroup with severe CHI involving injury to the frontal lobe would have the poorest WM.

4. Evaluate age at injury and time since injury as predictors of WM age percentiles. We hypothesized that an earlier age at injury and a shorter time since injury would be associated with poorer WM.

5. Evaluate WM components in relation to CHI severity and biological and developmental moderators. We hypothesized that (a) severe CHI would be associated with problems in WM components, whereas milder forms of injury would be associated with selective or no component deficits, and (b) severe CHI involving injury to the frontal lobe, an earlier age at injury, and a shorter time since injury would be associated with poorer component WM performance.

METHOD

Participants

The study sample consisted of 126 school-age children and adolescents (76 boys, 50 girls) who had sustained a CHI requiring hospital admission. We recruited participants from both research studies and clinical sources at The Hospital for Sick Children in Toronto, Canada. Four sets of siblings were included in the study. Inclusion–exclusion criteria were established from medical records and IQ tests. Included participants had a single head injury at least 1 year before testing and Verbal Performance IQ scores above 70 on a standard test of intelligence (Wechsler, 1974, 1991). Exclusion criteria were preexisting neurologic disorder associated with cerebral dysfunction and/or cognitive deficit (e.g., birth anoxia, preexisting seizures), severe preexisting psychiatric disorder (e.g., autism), or inflicted or gunshot injury. Because of the difficulty in establishing a consistent diagnosis of premorbid attention or learning disorders in this retrospective cohort, these conditions were not explicitly excluded.

Injury severity grouping. On the basis of nonparalyzed coma scale rating, length of loss or disruption of consciousness, neurosurgical intervention, and neuroimaging findings, participants were divided into three CHI severity groups: *mild* ($N = 40$), *moderate* ($N = 46$), and *severe* ($N = 40$). Coma scale ratings were taken as the lowest assigned score in the ambulance or on admission to the Emergency Room of the first hospital visited. We used the Glasgow Coma Scale (Teasdale & Jennett, 1974) for participants who were injured at or after 2 years of age, and the Children's Modified Glasgow Coma Score (Raimondi & Hirschauer, 1984) for participants who were injured under the age of 2 years. Length of loss or disruption of consciousness was recorded in minutes or days. The mild group had a coma score of 13 to 15 ($M = 14.54$, $SD = 0.76$), loss or disruption of consciousness of less than 15 min, no neurosurgical intervention, and negative neuroimaging findings aside from any linear skull fracture. The moderate group included participants who either had a coma score of 9 to 12 with a loss or disruption of consciousness and positive or negative neuroimaging findings, or had a coma score greater than 12 with positive neuroimaging findings, neurosurgical intervention, or both

($M = 12.76$, $SD = 2.05$). The severe group had a coma score of 3 to 8 ($M = 5.98$, $SD = 1.64$) and a loss or disruption of consciousness of more than 15 min. Most of the severe injuries involved focal contusions, diffuse axonal injury, or both. Table 1 outlines the demographic characteristics of the sample. The CHI severity groups did not differ in age at test, age at injury, or time since injury.

Frontal injury grouping. Participants were also assigned a *frontal* score on the basis of available medical data and neuroimaging findings. By definition, all members of the mild group had a frontal score of 0. Those in the moderate or severe groups with positive findings of frontal lobe pathology confirmed by neuroimaging or at neurosurgery were assigned a score of 1; otherwise, they received a score of 0. This assignment produced subsets of the moderate and severe CHI severity groups: *frontal-moderate* ($N = 24$), *frontal-severe* ($N = 23$), *nonfrontal-moderate* ($N = 22$), and *nonfrontal-severe* ($N = 17$). The frontal subsets did not differ in age at test, age at injury, or time since injury (see Table 1 for means and standard deviations). The specificity of frontal injury (vis-à-vis other focal brain injuries) could not be addressed because the moderate and severe injuries without evidence of frontal injury either had no other focal injury or had a diversely located range of bleeds and contusions.

Procedure

In a quiet room, participants were individually administered the Recognition Memory Test (Goldman, Fristoe, & Woodcock, 1974), an auditory-verbal WM task that involves judgments about the prior occurrence of target words. The task consisted of 110 words, divided into five blocks of 22 words, which had been drawn randomly from a pool of 1,200 words selected on the basis of familiarity, concreteness, common length, and syllable structure (Goldman et al., 1974). A standard training section introduced the task and provided some practice. The test was then administered in accordance with the instructions provided in the test manual (including the discontinue criteria). The test words were presented aurally by prerecorded tape. Each test word occurred twice within a block, and no word occurred in more than one block. The separation of first and second presentations of a word ranged from no intervening words (during a 3-sec time period) to eight intervening words (during a 24-sec time period). There were 6 items for each level of word separation, except for items with 4 intervening words, for which there were 7. Participants were asked to respond to each word by indicating whether or not it had been heard previously in the list. The task required participants to retain incoming verbal information over short time periods, to perform a simple computational operation of comparing new to old information, and to remember the updated memory register. These active and prospective features identify the task as one of verbal WM.

TABLE 1
Demographic Characteristics of the Closed Head Injury Sample

Group	N	Coma Score		Age at Test		Age at Injury		Time Since Injury	
		M	SD	M	SD	M	SD	M	SD
Severity groups									
Mild	40	14.54	0.76	10.94	3.19	7.29	3.91	3.66	1.70
Moderate	46	12.76	2.05	10.31	3.35	7.31	3.80	3.00	1.62
Severe	40	5.98	1.64	10.85	3.15	7.21	3.70	3.64	1.95
Frontal subsets									
Frontal–moderate	24	13.04	2.05	10.88	3.70	8.30	3.85	2.57	1.30
Frontal–severe	23	5.83	1.85	10.89	3.42	7.35	4.10	3.54	2.11
Nonfrontal–moderate	22	12.45	2.04	9.69	2.88	6.22	3.50	3.47	1.82
Nonfrontal–severe	17	6.18	1.33	10.80	2.86	7.03	3.20	3.77	1.76

Four WM scores were derived from task performance: *age percentile, task maintenance, item maintenance,* and *load.* Age percentiles were calculated using the standardized tables provided in the test manual (Goldman et al., 1974). Task maintenance is the ability to hold the task requirements over time from the first to the last set of items. It was calculated as a difference score of the raw total in Block 5 (out of 22) from the raw total in Block 1 (out of 22). Task maintenance scores ranged from –22 to 22, with a score of 0 reflecting perfect maintenance. Item maintenance is the ability to hold (e.g., via rehearsal) and retrieve task items for cognitive performance. It was defined in this study as the sum of raw scores on trials in which the second presentation of the word occurred after 6, 7, or 8 intervening words (i.e., those with a high item maintenance demand). Because there were 6 items at each word separation level, item maintenance scores ranged from 0 to 18. Load is the amount of information that can be reliably stored during WM processing, therefore measuring online WM capacity. Load was operationally defined as the highest number of intervening words at which perfect performance was achieved. Load scores ranged from 0 to 8.

RESULTS

Age Percentiles

Score distribution. The distribution of WM age percentiles for the entire sample showed a significant positive skew, $D(126) = .125, p < .001$. Figure 1 displays the distribution of scores and Table 2 contains the mean and standard devia-

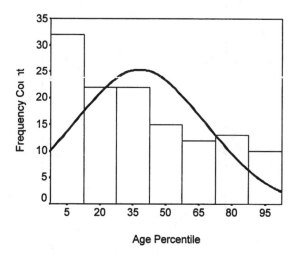

FIGURE 1   Distribution of WM age percentiles in the CHI sample.

TABLE 2
Working Memory Scores

Group	N	Age Percentile		Task Maintenance		Item Maintenance		Load	
		M	SD	M	SD	M	SD	M	SD
Entire sample	126	38.02	29.69	1.66	1.90	13.54	3.41	5.40	2.93
Severity groups									
Mild	40	46.13	32.13	1.05	1.58	14.25	2.76	5.80	2.86
Moderate	46	39.72	27.53	1.87	2.18	13.76	3.67	5.48	3.05
Severe	40	27.98	27.29	2.03	1.73	12.58	3.53	4.93	2.88
Frontal subsets									
Frontal–moderate	24	45.92	27.72	1.04	1.57	14.33	4.33	6.08	2.64
Frontal–severe	23	30.70	28.96	1.83	1.75	13.17	3.34	5.22	3.00
Nonfrontal–moderate	22	32.95	26.28	2.77	2.41	13.14	2.75	4.82	3.38
Nonfrontal–severe	17	24.29	25.22	2.29	1.72	11.76	3.72	4.53	2.74

tion of the sample. In the long term after a CHI, children had verbal WM scores that were nonnormally distributed, with scores skewed toward the lower end of the distribution.

CHI severity.   We also examined the WM age percentile distributions of each CHI severity group. The moderate and severe groups showed significant positive skews: $D(46) = .154, p < .01$ and $D(40) = .196, p < .005$, respectively (see Figure 2). The mild group was normally distributed, although quite variable with scores ranging from the 1st to the 99th percentile. We reviewed the medical histories of the mild CHI children who had scores below the 5th percentile ($n = 8$); none had any reported premorbid attention or learning disorders.

An analysis of variance (ANOVA) assessing CHI severity group differences in age percentiles was significant, $F(2, 123) = 4.04, p < .05$ (see Table 2 for CHI severity group means and standard deviations). Tukey pairwise comparisons indicated that the severe group scored significantly below the mild group. The moderate group did not differ from either the severe or the mild group. Inspection of the medians for the moderate and severe groups (30.5 and 17.5, respectively) highlights the extent to which impaired WM performance was associated with both moderate and severe CHI.

In comparison to the population mean (i.e., the 50th percentile), the severe and moderate groups were significantly below average, $t(39) = -5.11, p < .001$ and $t(45) = -2.53, p < .05$, respectively. The mild group did not differ from the normative.

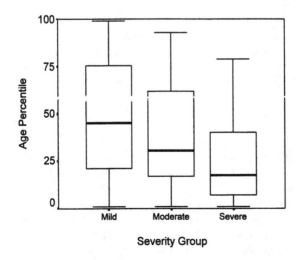

FIGURE 2   Box plots of WM age percentiles for each CHI severity group.

Biological moderators.   Using the frontal subsets of the sample, we performed a two-way ANOVA of WM age percentile, with severity group and frontal score as the between-subjects variables. The interaction of severity group and frontal score was not significant. Injury to the frontal lobe did not moderate severity effects on overall verbal WM performance.

Developmental moderators.   We used multiple regression models to predict WM age percentiles from age at injury and time since injury within each CHI severity group. None of the models was significant. Developmental variables did not moderate overall verbal WM performance after childhood CHI.

WM Components

CHI severity.   ANCOVAs were used to evaluate CHI severity group differences in task maintenance, item maintenance, and load, with age at test as a covariate because scores were not age adjusted. All ANCOVAs were significant: task maintenance, $F(3, 122) = 3.44$, $p < .05$; item maintenance, $F(3, 122) = 7.74$, $p < .001$; load, $F(3, 122) = 3.74$, $p < .05$, and showed age at test effects: task maintenance, $F(1, 122) = 3.79$, $p < .06$; item maintenance, $F(1, 122) = 17.24$, $p < .001$; load: $F(1, 122) = 9.27$, $p < .005$. There were severity effects for task maintenance, $F(2, 122) = 3.06$, $p < .06$, and item maintenance, $F(2, 122) = 3.17$, $p < .05$, but not load. Tukey pairwise comparisons showed that the severe group had significantly poorer task and item maintenance than the mild group. The moderate group did not differ from either the severe or the mild group.

Biological moderators.   Using the frontal subsets, we performed two-way ANOVAs of the three WM components, with severity group and frontal score as the between-subjects variables. As was the case with overall WM performance, the interaction of severity group and frontal score was not significant for any WM component.

Developmental moderators.   Using multiple regression models within each CHI severity group, we predicted task maintenance, item maintenance, and load from age at injury and time since injury. None of the models predicting task maintenance was significant. Within the moderate group, a younger age at injury and a shorter time since injury predicted poorer item maintenance and load, $F(2, 43) = 7.82$, $p < .005$, adjusted $R^2 = .23$ and $F(2, 43) = 9.43$, $p < .001$, adjusted $R^2 = .27$, respectively. The item maintenance and load models for the mild and severe groups were not significant. Developmental variables were predictive of WM component processes after CHI of moderate severity.

DISCUSSION

CHI often results in neuropsychological sequelae that persist well into the recovery period. Memory impairment is consistently part of the cognitive morbidity associated with childhood CHI. This study supports recent demonstrations of verbal WM deficits after childhood CHI (Levin et al., 2002; Proctor et al., 2000), and adds information about CHI severity and moderating factors with a sufficiently large sample tested well into the chronic recovery phase.

In children, severity of CHI is a powerful determinant of verbal WM, even many years after the insult. Severe CHI continues to be associated with significant overall WM impairment, as well as deficits in component processes of WM. Moderate CHI is also associated with impaired WM performance, although to a lesser extent than severe CHI. Mild CHI spares verbal WM on a groupwise basis, although some individuals show significant WM impairment when compared to a normative group. In this subset of the mild CHI group, there were no parent reports of premorbid attention or learning problems. Nonetheless, these individuals might have had poorer WM outcome related to the biological impact of their injury not demonstrated on current structural neuroimaging modalities. Adults with CHI of varying severity recruit more regionally dispersed frontal brain regions than controls while performing WM tasks (Christodoulou et al., 2001), and, even though task performance is similar to controls after mild CHI, brain activation patterns differ (McAllister et al., 2001). Future studies should investigate the anatomical microstructure and brain activation patterns after childhood CHI to better understand the sources of individual variability in WM function within and across severity groups.

Moderator variables were evaluated because the relation between CHI severity and WM is imperfect. Frontal lobe pathology did not account for variability in verbal WM performance. There may be several reasons for this null result. In adults, the manipulation component of WM has the strongest association with frontal lesions (Postle et al., 1999). The effects of frontal pathology might, therefore, have been more evident in WM measures involving a heavier manipulation component, rather than maintenance and load components. The coding used here identified the presence or absence of frontal lesions, but did not account for extrafrontal lesions. Moreover, our coding did not identify damage according to subregions of the frontal lobe. WM function has been linked to particular subdivisions of the prefrontal cortex (Bunge, Ochsner, Desmond, Glover, & Gabrieli, 2001; D'Esposito, Postle, Ballard, & Lease, 1999; Fletcher & Henson, 2001; Petrides, Alivisatos, Meyer, & Evans, 1993), particularly in the dorsolateral area. Future studies using quantitative volumetric analysis of brain lesions in conjunction with cognitive measures would undoubtedly increase the specificity of outcome in WM function associated with the location and extent of frontal lobe injury.

Developmental moderator variables were not predictive of overall WM level many years after mild or severe childhood CHI. Our results suggest that the biological impact of a severe CHI overrides the moderating effects of age and time variables. For injuries of moderate severity, however, WM function does appear to be related to the age at which the injury was sustained, as well as the time that has elapsed since the injury. These data are consistent with an emerging body of evidence showing that early CHI is a significant risk factor for poor long-term cognitive outcome (Anderson & Moore, 1995; Koskiniemi, Kyykka, Nybo, & Jarho, 1995; Kriel, Krach, & Panser, 1989; Slomine et al., 2002; Taylor & Alden, 1997; Wrightson, McGinn, & Gronwall, 1995; Yeates, 2000). Poor WM outcome after early childhood CHI could be a result of developmental instability, or the derailing of normal development because of abnormal influences, of which CHI is one (Yeo, Hill, Campbell, Vigil, & Brooks, 2000). Higher order abilities, such as a theory of mind, are dependent on age-related improvement in core cognitive resources, including WM (Carlson & Moses, 2001). An early age at injury and associated WM impairments, then, may underlie various forms of executive dysfunction exhibited after childhood CHI (e.g., metacognition, Dennis, Barnes, Donnelly, Wilkinson, & Humphreys, 1996; attentional–inhibitory control, Dennis, Guger, Roncadin, Barnes, & Schachar, 2001). Prospective studies across developmental stages could elucidate the reciprocal influences that core cognitive resources, including WM, exert on each other and higher order abilities.

Premorbid history and postinjury environment are also important determinants of recovery after CHI (Satz, Zaucha, McCleary, Light, & Asarnow, 1997; Yeates et al., 1997), although this study did not evaluate these factors. Some of the subjects at the lower end of the distributions of our mild and moderate CHI groups might represent variation in these factors, rather than direct consequences of the CHI. Family distress and burden, for example, can increase the likelihood of poor outcome (Taylor & Alden, 1997; Taylor et al., 1995). Prospective studies may help to clarify whether or not some of the variability in verbal WM outcome after childhood CHI can be explained by environmental factors.

We examined three WM components to better understand the nature of verbal WM impairment after childhood CHI. Task maintenance evaluates the extent to which response requirements are held and applied throughout the task. After a severe CHI, task maintenance is compromised. Performance on items requiring sustained activation (i.e., item maintenance) is also deficient after severe CHI relative to milder injuries. Poor WM performance after a severe CHI is, in part, attributable to impairments in the ability to maintain the task requirements and hold several items online to prepare for an upcoming response. WM deficits in children with severe CHI, then, might represent a compromise of general executive and attentional processes beyond those associated with using WM. Poor verbal WM after moderate CHI appears to reflect a more selective impairment in item-specific load and maintenance components of WM. In the current paradigm, mild CHI is not associated with component verbal WM deficits.

Several years beyond medical recovery, children with moderate or severe CHI have significant and persistent WM deficits related to holding verbal information online, limiting the computational workspace required for many cognitive tasks. Differential findings with load and maintenance aspects of WM are consistent with recent studies showing that, in recognition memory and WM span tasks, both resource sharing and a less rapid temporal decay improve developmentally (Barrouillet & Camos, 2001; Cowan, 1997). Injury severity plays a significant role in these deficits. In view of the importance of WM for academic function, such as mediating long-term memory for mathematical algorithms (Swanson & Sachse-Lee, 2001), the persistence of verbal WM deficits many years after moderate or severe CHI is likely related to the poor functional outcome in academic areas commonly associated with childhood CHI (Ewing-Cobbs et al., this issue).

ACKNOWLEDGMENTS

Supported in part by National Institute of Neurological Disorders and Stroke Grant 2R01NS21889–16 and by project grants from The Physicians' Services Incorporated and the Ontario Mental Health Foundation.

Some of the data were presented at the 28th annual meeting of the International Neuropsychological Society (Denver, CO, February 2000).

We thank Margaret Wilkinson for assistance with data collection and scoring and Laura Mansueti for assistance with manuscript preparation.

REFERENCES

Anderson, V., & Moore, C. (1995). Age at injury as a predictor of outcome following pediatric head injury: A longitudinal perspective. *Child Neuropsychology, 1,* 187–202.

Awh, E., Smith, E. E., & Jonides, J. (1995). Human rehearsal processes and the frontal lobes: PET evidence. In J. Grafman, K. J., Holyoak, & F. Boller (Eds.), *Annals of the New York Academy of Sciences: Vol. 769. Structure and functions of the human prefrontal cortex* (pp. 97–117). New York: New York Academy of Sciences.

Baddeley, A. D. (1986). *Working memory.* Oxford, England: Clarendon.

Barnes, M. A., & Dennis, M. (2001). Knowledge-based inferencing after childhood head injury. *Brain and Language, 76,* 253–265.

Barrouillet, P., & Camos, V. (2001). Developmental increase in working memory span: Resource sharing or temporal decay? *Journal of Memory and Language, 45,* 1–20.

Bjorklund, D. F., & Harnishfeger, K. K. (1990). The resources construct in cognitive development: Diverse sources of evidence and a theory of inefficient inhibition. *Developmental Review, 10,* 48–71.

Brookshire, B. L., Chapman, S. B., Song, J., & Levin, H. S. (2000). Cognitive and linguistic correlates of children's discourse after closed head injury: A three-year follow-up. *Journal of the International Neuropsychological Society, 6,* 741–751.

Bull, R., & Scerif, G. (2001). Executive functioning as a predictor of children's mathematical ability: Inhibition, switching, and working memory. *Developmental Neuropsychology, 19,* 273–293.

Bunge, S. A., Ochsner, K. N., Desmond, J. E., Glover, G. H., & Gabrieli, J. D. E. (2001). Prefrontal regions involved in keeping information in and out of mind. *Brain, 124,* 2074–2086.

Carlson, S. M., & Moses, L. J. (2001). Individual differences in inhibitory control and children's theory of mind. *Child Development, 72,* 1032–1053.

Case, R. (1985). *Intellectual development: Birth to adulthood.* New York: Academic.

Chadwick, O., Rutter, M., Shaffer, D., & Shrout, M. (1981). A prospective study of children with head injuries: II. Cognitive sequelae. *Psychological Medicine, 11,* 49–61.

Chapman, S. B., Culhane, K. A., Levin, H. S., Harward, H., Mendelsohn, D., Ewing-Cobbs, L., et al. (1992). Narrative discourse after closed head injury in children and adolescents. *Brain and Language, 43,* 42–65.

Cowan, N. (1997). The development of working memory. In N. Cowan & C. Hulme (Eds.), *The development of memory in childhood* (pp. 163–200). Hove, UK: Psychology.

Christodoulou, C., DeLuca, J., Ricker, J. H., Madigan, N. K., Bly, B. M., Lange, G., et al. (2001). Functional magnetic resonance imaging of working memory impairment after traumatic brain injury. *Journal of Neurology, Neurosurgery, and Psychiatry, 71,* 161–168.

Dennis, M. (1988). Language and the young damaged brain. In T. Boll & B. K. Bryant (Eds.), *Clinical neuropsychology and brain function: Research, measurement, and practice* (pp. 89–123). Washington, DC: American Psychological Association.

Dennis, M., & Barnes, M. A. (1990). Knowing the meaning, getting the point, bridging the gap, and carrying the message: Aspects of discourse following closed head injury in childhood and adolescence. *Brain and Language, 39,* 428–446.

Dennis, M., & Barnes, M. A. (2000). Speech acts after mild or severe childhood head injury. *Aphasiology, 14,* 391–405.

Dennis, M., & Barnes, M. A. (2001). Comparison of literal, inferential, and intentional text comprehension in children with mild or severe closed head injury. *Journal of Head Trauma Rehabilitation, 16,* 456–468.

Dennis, M., Barnes, M. A., Donnelly, R. E., Wilkinson, M., & Humphreys, R. P. (1996). Appraising and managing knowledge: Metacognitive skills after childhood head injury. *Developmental Neuropsychology, 12,* 77–103.

Dennis, M., Guger, S., Roncadin, C., Barnes, M., & Schachar, R. (2001). Attentional-inhibitory control and social-behavioral regulation after childhood closed head injury: Do biological, developmental, and recovery variables predict outcome? *Journal of the International Neuropsychological Society, 7,* 683–692.

D'Esposito, M., Postle, B. R., Ballard, D., & Lease, J. (1999). Maintenance versus manipulation of information held in working memory: An event-related fMRI study. *Brain and Cognition, 41,* 66–86.

Ewing-Cobbs, L., Barnes, M., Fletcher, J. M., Levin, H. S., Swank, P. R., & Song, J. (2004/this issue). Modeling of longitudinal academic achievement scores after pediatric traumatic brain injury. *Developmental Neuropsychology, 25,* 107–133.

Fay, G. C., Jaffe, K. M., Polissar, N. L., Liao, S., Rivara, J. B., & Martin, K. M. (1994). Outcome of pediatric traumatic brain injury at three years: A cohort study. *Archives of Physical Medicine and Rehabilitation, 75,* 733–741.

Fletcher, P. C. & Henson, R. N. A. (2001). Frontal lobes and human memory. *Brain, 124,* 849–881.

Gathercole, S. E., & Pickering, S. J. (2000). Working memory deficits in children with low achievements in the national curriculum at 7 years of age. *British Journal of Educational Psychology, 70,* 177–194.

Goldman, R., Fristoe, M., & Woodcock, R. (1974). *Technical manual for Goldman-Fristoe-Woodcock Auditory Skills Test Battery.* Circle Pines, MN: American Guidance Service.

Hanten, G., Levin, H. S., & Song, J. X. (1999). Working memory and metacognition in sentence comprehension by severely head-injured children: A preliminary study. *Developmental Neuropsychology, 16,* 393–414.

Hulme, C., & Roodenrys, S. (1995). Practitioner review: Verbal working memory development and its disorders. *Journal of Child Psychology and Psychiatry, 36,* 373–398.

Koskiniemi, M., Kyykka, T., Nybo, T., & Jarho, L. (1995). Long-term outcome after severe brain injury in preschoolers is worse than expected. *Archives of Pediatric Adolescent Medicine, 149,* 249–254.

Kriel, R. L., Krach, L. E., & Panser, L. A. (1989). Closed head injury: Comparison of children younger and older than 6 years of age. *Pediatric Neurology, 5,* 296–300.

Levin, H. S., Eisenberg, H. M., Wigg, N. R., & Kobayashi, K. (1982). Memory and intellectual ability after head injury in children and adolescents. *Neurosurgery, 11,* 668–673.

Levin, H. S., Fletcher, J. M., Kusnerik, L., Kufera, J., Lilly, M. A., Duffy, F. F., et al. (1996). Semantic memory following pediatric head injury: Relationship to age, severity of injury, and MRI. *Cortex, 32,* 461–478.

Levin, H. S., Hanten, G., Chang, C., Zhang, L., Schachar, R., Ewing-Cobbs, L., et al. (2002). Working memory after traumatic brain injury in children. *Annals of Neurology, 52,* 82–88.

Levin, H. S., High, W. M., Jr., Ewing-Cobbs, L., Fletcher, J. M., Eisenberg, H. M., Miner, M. E., et al. (1988). Memory functioning during the first year after closed head injury in children and adolescents. *Neurosurgery, 22,* 1043–1052.

Logie, R. H. (1996). The seven ages of working memory. In J. T. E. Richardson, R. W. Engle, L. Hasher, R. H. Logie, E. R. Stoltzfus, & R. T. Zacks (Eds.), *Working memory and human cognition* (pp. 31–65). New York: Oxford University.

MacKenzie, J. D., Siddiqi, F., Babb, J. S., Bagley, L. J., Mannon, L. J., Sinson, G. P., et al. (2002). Brain atrophy in mild or moderate traumatic brain injury: A longitudinal quantitative analysis. *American Journal of Neuroradiology, 23,* 1509–1515.

McAllister, T. W., Sparling, M. B., Flashman, L. A., Guerin, S. J., Mamourian, A. C., & Saykin, A. J. (2001). Differential working memory load effects after mild traumatic brain injury. *NeuroImage, 14,* 1004–1012.

Mendelsohn, D., Levin, H. S., Bruce, D., Lilly, M., Harward, H., Culhane, K. A., et al. (1992). Late MRI after head injury in children: Relationship to clinical features and outcome. *Child Nervous System, 8,* 445–452.

Montgomery, J. W. (1995). Sentence comprehension in children with specific language impairment: The role of phonological working memory. *Journal of Speech and Hearing Research, 33,* 187–199.

Palmer, H. M., & McDonald, S. (2000). The role of frontal and temporal lobe processes in prospective remembering. *Brain and Cognition, 44,* 103–107.

Passolunghi, M. C., & Siegel, L. S. (2001). Short-term memory, working memory, and inhibitory control in children with difficulties in arithmetic problem solving. *Journal of Experimental Child Psychology, 80,* 44–57.

Petrides, M. (2000). Dissociable roles of mid-dorsolateral prefrontal and anterior inferotemporal cortex in visual working memory. *The Journal of Neuroscience, 20,* 7496–7503.

Petrides, M., Alivisatos, B., Meyer, E., & Evans, A. C. (1993). Functional activation of the human frontal cortex during the performance of verbal working memory tasks. *Proceedings of the National Academy of Sciences, 90,* 878–882.

Postle, B. R., Berger, J. S., & D'Esposito, M. (1999). Functional neuroanatomical double-dissociation of mnemonic and executive control processes contributing to working memory performance. *Proceedings of the National Academy of Sciences, 96,* 12959–12964.

Proctor, A., Wilson, B., Sanchez, C., & Wesley, E. (2000). Executive function and verbal working memory in adolescents with closed head injury (CHI). *Brain Injury, 14,* 633–647.

Raimondi, A. J., & Hirschauer, J. (1984). Head injury in the infant and toddler. *Child's Brain, 11,* 12–35.

Richardson, J. T. E. (1996). Evolving concepts of working memory. In J. T. E. Richardson, R. W. Engle, L. Hasher, R. H. Logie, E. R. Stoltzfus, & R. T. Zacks (Eds.), *Working memory and human cognition* (pp. 3–30). New York: Oxford University.

Roman, M. J., Delis, D. C., Willerman, L., Magulac, M., Demadura, T. L. de la Pena, J. L., et al. (1998). Impact of pediatric traumatic brain injury on components of verbal memory. *Journal of Clinical and Experimental Neuropsychology, 20,* 245–258.

Roncadin, C., Pascual-Leone, J., Rich, J. B., & Dennis, M. (2003). *Developmental relations between working memory and inhibitory control.* Manuscript submitted for publication.

Satz, P., Zaucha, K., McCleary, C., Light, R., & Asarnow, R. (1997). Mild head injury in children and adolescents: A review of studies (1970–1995). *Psychological Bulletin, 122,* 107–131.

Slomine, B. S., Gerring, J. P., Grados, M. A., Vasa, R., Brady, K. D., Christensen, J. R., et al. (2002). Performance on measures of 'executive function' following pediatric traumatic brain injury. *Brain Injury, 16,* 759–772.

Swanson, H. L. (1993). Working memory and learning disability subgroups. *Journal of Experimental Child Psychology, 56,* 87–114.

Swanson, H. L., & Sachse-Lee, C. (2001). Mathematical problem solving and working memory in children with learning disabilities: Both executive and phonological processes are important. *Journal of Experimental Child Psychology, 79,* 294–321.

Taylor, H. G., & Alden, J. (1997). Age-related differences in outcomes following childhood brain insults: An introduction and overview. *Journal of the International Neuropsychological Society, 3,* 555–567.

Taylor, H. G., Drotar, D., Wade, S., Yeates, K. O., Stancin, T., & Klein, S. (1995). Recovery from traumatic brain injury in children: The importance of the family. In S. H. Broman & M. E. Michel (Eds.), *Traumatic head injury in children* (pp. 188–218). New York: Oxford University.

Teasdale, G., & Jennett, B. (1974). Assessment of coma and impaired consciousness. *Lancet, 2,* 81–84.

Turkstra, L. S., & Holland, A. L. (1998). Assessment of syntax after adolescent brain injury: Effects of memory on test performance. *Journal of Speech and Language Hearing Research, 41,* 137–149.

Verger, K., Junque, C., Jurado, M. A., Tresserras, P., Bartumeus, F., Nogues, P., et al. (2000). Age effects on long-term neuropsychological outcome in pediatric traumatic brain injury. *Brain Injury, 14,* 495–503.

Wechsler, D. (1974). *Wechsler Intelligence Scale for Children-Revised.* New York: The Psychological Corporation.

Wechsler, D. (1991). *Wechsler Intelligence Scale for Children-Third Edition.* New York: The Psychological Corporation.

Wrightson, P., McGinn, V., & Gronwall, D. (1995). Mild head injury in preschool children: Evidence that it can be associated with a persisting cognitive defect. *Journal of Neurology, Neurosurgery, and Psychiatry, 59,* 375–380.

Yeates, K. O. (2000). Closed-head injury. In K. O. Yeates, M. D. Ris, & H. G. Taylor (Eds.), *Pediatric neuropsychology: Research, theory, and practice* (pp. 92–116). New York: Guilford.

Yeates, K. O., Blumenstein, E., Patterson, C. M., & Delis, D. C. (1995). Verbal learning and memory following pediatric closed-head injury. *Journal of the International Neuropsychological Society, 1,* 78–87.

Yeates, K. O., Taylor, H. G., Drotar, D., Wade, S., Klein, S., Stancin, T., et al. (1997). Preinjury family environment as a determinant of recovery from traumatic brain injuries in school-age children. *Journal of the International Neuropsychological Society, 3,* 617–630.

Yeo, R. A., Hill, D., Campbell, R., Vigil, J., & Brooks, W. M. (2000). Developmental instability and working memory ability in children: A magnetic resonance spectroscopy investigation. *Developmental Neuropsychology, 17,* 143–159.

DEVELOPMENTAL NEUROPSYCHOLOGY, 25(1&2), 37–60

Discourse Macrolevel Processing After Severe Pediatric Traumatic Brain Injury

Sandra Bond Chapman and Garen Sparks
Center for BrainHealth
The University of Texas at Dallas

Harvey S. Levin
Cognitive Neuroscience Laboratory
Departments of Physical Medicine and Rehabilitation,
Neurosurgery, and Psychiatry and Behavioral Sciences
Baylor College of Medicine
Houston, TX

Maureen Dennis and Caroline Roncadin
Department of Psychology
Hospital for Sick Children
Toronto, Ontario, Canada

Lifang Zhang
Cognitive Neuroscience Laboratory
Department of Physical Medicine and Rehabilitation
Baylor College of Medicine
Houston, TX

James Song
Department of Biometry
Bayer Pharmaceuticals
West Haven, CT

Requests for reprints should be sent to Sandra Bond Chapman, Center for BrainHealth, The University of Texas at Dallas, 1966 Inwood Road, Dallas, TX 75235. E-mail: schapman@utdallas.edu

The purpose of this study was to determine if discourse macrolevel processing abilities differed between children with severe traumatic brain injury (TBI) at least 2 years postinjury and typically developing children. Twenty-three children had sustained a severe TBI either before the age of 8 ($n = 10$) or after the age of 8 ($n = 13$). The remaining 32 children composed a control group of typically developing peers. The groups' summaries and interpretive lesson statements were analyzed according to reduction and transformation of narrative text information. Compared to the control group, the TBI group condensed the original text information to a similar extent. However, the TBI group produced significantly less transformed information during their summaries, especially those children who sustained early injuries. The TBI and control groups did not significantly differ in their production of interpretive lesson statements. In terms of related skills, discourse macrolevel summarization ability was significantly related to problem solving but not to lexical or sentence level language skills or memory. Children who sustain a severe TBI early in childhood are at an increased risk for persisting deficits in higher level discourse abilities, results that have implications for academic success and therapeutic practices.

One of the most formidable tasks to improving the long-term cognitive-linguistic outcome in pediatric brain injury is to better understand the paradox of recovery for many of these children. For example, why is it that many children with severe brain injury show remarkable recovery on standardized language and cognitive measures, yet fail in the classroom? Whereas the answer to this quandary is certainly multifaceted, new evidence suggests that discourse macrolevel deficits may contribute to learning difficulties that persist at later stages post brain injury. This study examines discourse macrolevel abilities in children with severe traumatic brain injury (TBI) in relation to the moderating effect of age at injury.

DISCOURSE MACROLEVEL PROCESSING

Definition

Discourse macrolevel processing is conceptualized as extracting the most important information from connected language (Ulatowska & Chapman, 1994; van Dijk, 1995). Measures of macrolevel processing are those that require processes of reduction and transformation of information while preserving the central meaning. Types of macrolevel texts include summaries, main ideas, outlines, titles, and interpretative statements. These texts are shorter versions of the original discourse text, recursively conveying the same general meaning but containing less detail (van Dijk, 1995). Discourse macrolevel processing is contrasted with microlevel processing, in which the focus is on the isolated details, number of words and word types, and grammatical proficiency in conveying information.

Development

The cognitive abilities underlying the development of discourse macrolevel processing have been classified as executive functions (Brown & Day, 1983; Chapman, Levin, & Lawyer, 1999). These executive functions include processes such as judgment and problem solving (involved in sorting information according to importance), manipulating information in working memory, selective retrieval of important information from memory, and inhibition of less important or irrelevant details. The linguistic prerequisites of discourse macrolevel processing include comprehension of the discourse content, adequate vocabulary skills, and syntactic proficiency to convey the ideas. High-level vocabulary skills and the use of more complex syntactic structures have also been associated with conveying information at more generalized levels as required in macrolevel texts (Johnson, 1983; Ulatowska & Chapman, 1994). Pediatric TBI has been associated with impairments in all of these cognitive and linguistic domains (Levin, Ewing-Cobbs, & Eisenberg, 1995).

The majority of studies on the summary skills focus on normally developing children and show that macrolevel processing becomes refined with increasing age (Brown & Day, 1983; Johnson, 1983; Kinnunen & Vauras, 1995; Revelle, Wellman, & Karabenick, 1985; Vauras, Kinnunen, & Kuusela, 1994). When elementary school-age children (first through fifth grade) summarize information, they rely predominantly on the strategy of simple deletion of less important details with retention of important information. More mature summarizers, typically high school and college age, combine ideas across paragraphs and transform information into more generalized–transformed statements. As a result, they are able to convey more information in fewer words when compared to younger children (Brown, Day, & Jones, 1983). Nonetheless, even elementary school age children (6 to 10 years of age) use transformational strategies in summaries approximately 30% of the time as compared to a sixty percent ratio in college students when the content is within their knowledge base (Johnson, 1983).

Discourse Macrolevel Abilities in Children With TBI

Studies of macrolevel processing have served to elucidate the dissociations that can occur between macro and microlevel processing in adult populations (Chapman, Ulatowska, et al., 1997; Chapman, Ulatowska, King, Johnson, & McIntire, 1995; Chapman et al., in press; Ulatowska & Chapman, 1994). For example, patients with aphasia and relatively intact cognition exhibit preserved macrolevel processing but marked disruption in microlevel details.

Studies of macrolevel processing in children have emerged to examine the full scope of cognitive-communicative problems in children with TBI, which has gone unidentified with the use of standardized cognitive and linguistic tests (Chadwick, Rutter, Brown, Shaffer, & Traub, 1981; Chapman, Levin, & Lawyer, 1999; Levin

& Eisenberg, 1979). New evidence suggests that discourse macrolevel processing may be particularly vulnerable to the effects of severe TBI, especially the earlier the injury, and recovers slower than microlevel abilities (Brookshire, Chapman, Song, & Levin, 2000; Chapman et al., 1992; Chapman et al., 1998; Chapman et al., 2001; Chapman, Watkins, et al., 1997; Dennis, Barnes, Donnelly, Wilkinson, & Humphreys, 1996; Dennis, Barnes, Wilkinson, & Humphreys, 1998; Dennis, Guger, Roncadin, Barnes, Schacter, 2001; Dennis, Purvis, Barnes, Wilkinson, & Winner, 2001; Yorkston, Jaffe, Polissar, Liao, & Fay, 1997). Specifically, children with severe TBI show a marked reduction in recall of the gist information and on formulating a synthesized, interpretative statement (Chapman, Watkins, et al., 1997), although they may remember a great deal of the isolated facts, depending on the task demand on memory (Chapman et al., 1992; Chapman et al., 1998; Chapman et al., 1999).

Limitations in Macrolevel Discourse Processing Research

There are two major limitations in previous research concerning macrolevel discourse processing in pediatric TBI. First, the discourse tasks were not specifically designed to require macrolevel processing. For example, the discourse tasks asked for verbal and written retells rather than summaries (Brookshire et al., 2000; Chapman et al., 1992; Chapman et al., 1998; Chapman, Levin, Matejka, Harward, & Kufera, 1995; Chapman, Watkins, et al., 1997; Yorkston, et al., 1997; Yorkston, Jaffe, Liao, & Polissar, 1999). Second, the discourse tasks utilized brief narrative texts that placed minimal demands on condensing information (Ulatowska & Chapman, 1994). In fact, short texts are harder to reduce and transform because the information is already condensed.

It remains unclear whether children with severe brain injury fail to convey the most important, macrolevel meaning due to an inability to distinguish the most important points from the details. Alternatively, the reduced expression of important information may result from processing overload on tasks that emphasize the recall of details. Our team has speculated that children with brain injury may focus on the microdetails at the expense of macrolevel processing (Chapman et al., 1999). Because facility in macrolevel processing is related to learning achievement in the classroom setting (Kinnunen & Vauras, 1995), identification of poor discourse macrolevel processing by children with TBI could serve as a useful diagnostic and intervention guideline at subsequent, long-term recovery intervals (Johnson, 1983; Malone & Mastropieri, 1992; Stein & Kirby, 1992; Ulatowska & Chapman, 1994).

Purpose of Study

The primary purpose of this study was to determine the long-term consequences of severe TBI in childhood on discourse macrolevel processing as compared to typically developing peers through the elicitation of a summary and a lesson statement after listening to a narrative. A secondary goal was to explore the moderating effects of age at injury on discourse macrolevel processing. Additionally, we examined the relations between discourse macrolevel processing and performance on related cognitive and linguistic measures.

METHODS

Participants

Fifty-five children, ages 7 to 14 years of age at the time of testing, participated in this study. The participants were recruited from a larger research project examining cognitive and linguistic recovery after brain injury. Twenty-three of the children suffered severe brain injuries at least 2 years prior to testing and 32 were typically developing children.

Children with TBI were eligible for inclusion according to the following criteria: (a) TBI requiring hospitalization at least 2 years prior to assessment; (b) case history evidence that the injury resulted from a nonpenetrating head trauma, for example, motor-vehicle collision, or blow to the head; (c) documentation that injury was severe as established by a Glasgow Coma Scale (GCS; Teasdale & Jennett, 1974) score of 3 to 8; (d) age 7 through 14 years at time of assessment; and (e) English as the primary language of at least one of the child's caregivers. Exclusion criteria for the study included (a) a prior history of neurologic or psychiatric disorder, (b) grade failure or previous diagnosis of learning disability or mental deficiency, (c) evidence of child abuse, and (d) a previous head injury resulting in hospitalization. Global outcome, assessed using a modified Glasgow Outcome Scale (Jennett & Bond, 1975) revealed that approximately 35% of the TBI group made a good recovery; however, almost 61% of these children were judged to have moderate disability.

To examine age at injury effects on discourse macrolevel processing, the TBI group was divided into two groups, that is, an early injury group consisting of children injured before 8 years of age and a late injury group consisting of children injured after 8 years. The cutoff of age 8 years was selected primarily because this is the age when summarization ability is emerging. Recent evidence suggests that children with traumatic brain injuries occurring prior to or during cognitive skill development are more vulnerable than when the injury occurs after the skill is well-developed (Ewing-Cobbs, Levin, Eisenberg, & Fletcher, 1987).

Table 1 summarizes demographic and clinical features of the two groups. Univariate analyses revealed no significant differences for age at test and parental socioeconomic level as reflected by the parent's education. However, there was a significant difference in gender distribution between the control and TBI group (p

TABLE 1
Demographic and Clinical Features of the Control and Severe Childhood
Head Injury Groups

Variable	Control[a]	Severe[b]
Mean age at test (years)	11.70 (*SD* 2.77)	12.42 (*SD* 2.10)
Young (<8 years)		11.10 (*SD* 1.81) Range: 7.6–13.9
Old (>8 years)		13.44 (*SD* 1.74) Range: 11.2–14.0)
Mean age range since time of injury (years)		
Young (<8 years)		5.24 (*SD* 1.13) Range: 3.0–6.9
Old (>8 years)		3.64 (*SD* 0.83) Range: 2.6–5.8)
Mean parental education (years)	14.23 (*SD* 2.97)	13.30 (*SD* 2.15)
Gender		
Male	15	17
Female	17	6
Mechanism of injury		
Fall		1
Auto passenger		10
Motor vehicle–pedestrian		4
Bicycle		4
Motorcycle		1
Sports or play		3
Hit by falling object		0
Other		0
Glasgow Outcome Scale		
Good recovery		8
Moderate recovery		14
Information not available		1

[a]$N = 32$. [b]$N = 23$.

= 0.05), with the TBI group containing a larger proportion of males (control = 47%; TBI = 74%).

Narrative Stimuli

The experimental discourse stimuli involved a didactic long narrative entitled the "The Rich Man and the Shoemaker." This narrative was adopted from a second-grade reading text to ensure that the linguistic level was age appropriate (Appendix). The central meaning of "The Rich Man and the Shoemaker" is relevant to all ages because the story's actions convey a life-long lesson that "money does not necessarily bring happiness." Thus, the story's linguistic and conceptual complexity was appropriate for children ages seven years and older. The story consisted of two episodes (i.e., setting, action, resolution) conveyed through 45 sentences and

548 words. This relatively long story was chosen to discourage attempts at verbatim recall. The participants were instructed to condense the information.

Procedures

Participants were tested individually in a quiet room. Prior to hearing the narrative passage, the child was briefly familiarized with what it means to give a summary and a lesson. The examiner instructed the child to choose one of two familiar videocassette movie covers, either "The Beauty and the Beast" or "The Lion King." According to the child's preference, the examiner asked the child to listen carefully and then read the back of the video cover, after which, the examiner emphasized how much information was in the actual movie and how the summary on the video cover gave only the main events leaving out all the unimportant, extra details. The child was also told that the story taught an important life lesson. In a pilot testing, consisting of 10 controls and 9 TBI children, we found that all participants showed the ability to reduce the information in the form of a summary given specific examples. Several lesson examples, for the video story, were provided to ensure that the child understood the task. Several lessons were also given to illustrate to the child that there might be several ways to derive an appropriate interpretive lesson. Then the examiner told the child to listen carefully to a story, called "The Rich Man and the Shoemaker." The examiner reminded the child that he or she would not have to remember all the details of the story but just the main point from the story. Immediately after hearing the story, the child was asked to give a shortened version of the story in his or her own words. The child was told to include enough information so that the general meaning was clear and to leave out the less important details. The child was then asked to give a lesson that could be learned from the story. The child's summary and lesson responses were audiotaped and transcribed verbatim.

Linguistic and Cognitive Measures

To assess the relation of specific language and cognitive abilities to discourse macrolevel skills, performance on selected measures administered in the larger project were used. Cognitive measures of problem solving and memory and linguistic measures of vocabulary and sentence formulation were selected based on the literature that these domains are prerequisite to development of macrorules in summarizing texts (Brown & Day, 1983; Chapman et al., 1998; Stein & Kirby, 1992; Ulatowska & Chapman, 1994).

Problem solving was assessed using the raw score on the Block Design subtest from the Wechsler Abbreviated Scale for Intelligence (WASI; Wechsler, 1999). This test requires that participants recreate a three-dimensional block design provided by the examiner with a matching, two-dimensional block design using wooden blocks.

To address the potential role of memory deficits in summarizing a story, a test of verbal recall, the California Verbal Learning Test (CVLT)–Children's Versions (Delis, Kramer, Kaplan, & Ober, 1986) was given. The CVLT measures free recall of a 15-word list given in five consecutive trials. The sum of recall over all five trials was the memory measure (raw score) used in this study.

The Vocabulary subtest of the WASI (Wechsler, 1999) was administered and a raw score was computed. This test requires the child define a number of words increasing in complexity from concrete to more abstract. The raw score for the Formulated Sentences subtest of The Clinical Evaluation of Language Fundamentals (CELF; Semel, Wiig, & Secord, 1995) was used as a measure of lower-level, sentential language ability. As the name suggests, the subtest requires the child to verbally formulate sentences from words provided by the examiner. The provided words range from simple nouns (i.e., children), verbs (i.e., gave), and adjectives (i.e., younger) to more complex temporal (i.e., until, by the time) and causal (i.e., because, in spite of) phrases and relations.

Discourse Measures

The summary responses were analyzed using a systematic method developed by the first author based on the work of Kirby and colleagues (Kirby, 1988, 1991; Kirby & Cantwell, 1985; Kirby & Pedwell, 1991; Kirby & Probert, 1988) and from Kinnunen and Vauras (1995), and they were detailed in a scoring manual for our purposes. Each child's summary was divided into individual t units. A t unit is roughly equivalent to a sentence or a complete idea that can generally stand alone (Hunt, 1965). A t unit is defined as one independent clause and all the dependent clauses that modify it. The total number of t units in each child's summary was counted as a measure of amount of language used. Then each t unit was coded according to whether it was transformed or untransformed using the coding schema outlined in Table 2.

The score used to compare macrolevel discourse processing between the severe TBI and control group was the percentage of macrolevel t units contained within the summary productions. The percentage represented the total number of transformed t units (t units receiving a rating of 4–9; Table 2) divided by the total number of t units. The percent of t units transformed in the summary productions was used as a global index to distinguish between summaries that showed minimal transformation of the explicit information (t units rated as 1–3, Table 2) from those that demonstrated a modest use of macrolevel rules to condense information. Sample stories and scoring are shown in the Appendix.

The interpretative story lesson was evaluated using a rating scale ranging from 0 to 9 points. The scoring procedure was modified from work of Delis, Kramer, and Kaplan (1984) and has been used extensively by our team for over 12 years.

TABLE 2
Discourse Coding Schema for Transformation Analysis

Score	Level of Transformation	Description
0	Inappropriate inclusion of information	Incorrect, repetitious, unimportant information that is vaguely stated
1	Untransformed information: Copying or minimally paraphrasing original information	Unimportant information: Story details not necessary to convey central meaning
2		Important information: Vaguely stated
3		Important information: Verbatim or close semantic paraphrase of the story information
4	Transformed information: Combining explicit ideas into more concise and generalized statements	Important information: Transformed through inferencing, connecting information within an episode, but vaguely stated
6		Important information: Transformed through inferencing, connecting information within an episode
9		Important information: A generalized interpretation across the entire story content

The scale includes the components of concrete versus abstract, accuracy, and completeness of response. Sample responses and scoring are shown in Table 3.

To establish reliability of the analyses, 25% of the summaries and lessons were randomly selected and analyzed separately by two trained raters. Reliability scoring for the summary response yielded point-by-point interrater agreements of 92% for t units and 95% for transformed and untransformed units. Reliability scoring for the interpretative lesson response was 94%.

RESULTS

Statistical Analyses

A SAS procedure called GENMOD was used in modeling the summary task measures of (a) amount of information (i.e., number of t units) and (b) percent of information transformed in the summary productions. The GENMOD procedure uses a generalized estimating equation (GEE), which generates likelihood ratio chi-square values (Liang & Zeger, 1986). The SAS procedure of GENMOD was used because the outcome variables were not continuous, normally distributed

TABLE 3
Scoring of Lesson Transformation and Example Responses

Score	Level of Transformation	Examples
0	Incorrect concrete or incorrect abstract	Do not steal anyone's money
Untransformed information: Concrete		
1	Minimally correct concrete: Summary-like statement of an event in the story	The shoemaker should have found a better hiding spot for the money
2	Partially correct concrete: Only part of the lesson is given correctly, and the other part is omitted	The shoemaker should not have worried about money
3	Correct concrete: Complete moral that is tied to the text and is related specifically to the characters in the story	The shoemaker should have been happy with what he had and not worry about being rich
Transformed information: Abstract		
4	Minimally correct abstract: An attempt at generalization but incomplete, partially inaccurate, or not the expected main moral	Be yourself all the time, even if you do not have money
6	Partially correct abstract: Only part of the lesson is expressed abstractly and correctly and the remainder is omitted	Money is not the most important thing in the world
9	Correct abstract: Correct main moral, not specifically tied to the story characters, and generalized across the entire story based on real-life context	Being happy is better than being rich

measures. The outcome variable for percent of information transformed was divided into two categories. Specifically, a cutoff value of 20% was selected to divide the participants into either low transformers who used 20% or less transformed statements in their summaries or high transformers who used more than 20% transformed statements. These criteria were based on empirical evidence that children ages 6 to 10 years transform summary information at an approximate level of 30%. We chose a 20% cutoff to be on the conservative side. Injury and age at test were independent variables.

To determine age at injury effects after TBI on the ability to transform information in summaries, a lower value of 0% was established a priori based on our pilot data that few transformed statements were used by children with TBI. Thus the outcome variable for transformed statements was used to divide the TBI group into two groups—a no transformer group (0% transformed statements) and a transformer group (>0% transformed statements). The Fisher's Exact Test was adopted for this analysis, because 25% of the cells had expected counts less than 5. The younger age at injury group was defined as younger than 8 years old when they were injured ($n = 10$) and the older age at injury group was equal to or older than 8 years at the time of injury ($n = 13$). As stated earlier, this age split was based on empirical evidence that the age of 8 years is the age when summarization ability is emerging. Consequently, we hypothesized that this age may represent a period when children are more vulnerable to the negative effects of traumatic brain injury on the development of discourse summary skills (Ewing-Cobbs, Levin, Eisenberg, & Fletcher, 1987). The outcome variable for the lesson response divided the groups by a cutoff of 9 versus a rating of less than 9. A score of 9 represented an abstract, correct, and complete response. The same SAS procedure GENMOD was used in modeling this variable as described earlier. Spearman rank correlation coefficients were calculated to examine relations with a single macrolevel discourse score (i.e., percent of units transformed) to the two cognitive (Block Design and CVLT) and two linguistic measures (Vocabulary and CELF).

Summary Productions

Group effects.   The statistical analysis revealed a significant difference in the percent of transformed information in the summary productions between the TBI group and the control group, $\chi^2(1, N = 55) = 3.79, p = .05$. Compared to controls, the TBI group produced less transformed information in their summaries (see Figures 1 and 2). No significant age at test effects was found for transformed statements.

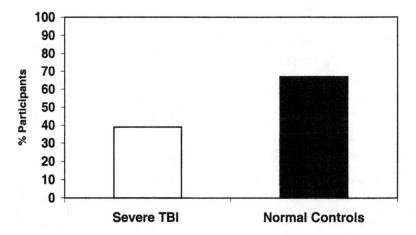

FIGURE 1   Percentage of control and severe TBI children whose summaries had greater than 20% transformed statements.

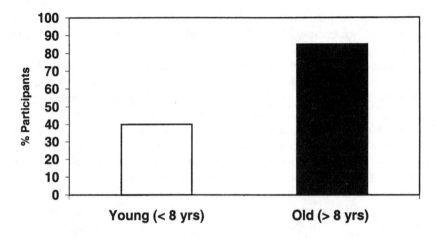

FIGURE 2   Percentage of severe TBI children (<8 years at injury) and severe TBI children (>8 years at injury) whose summaries contained transformed statements.

For the amount of language measure, there were no significant differences between the control and severe TBI groups. Both groups showed a similar degree of reduction in the amount of language used to give a summary of the original lengthy story containing 45 t units. There was a significant age at test effect, $\chi^2(1, N = 55) = 7.58$, $p = .006$, with older children using more t units.

For the interpretative lesson response, no significant difference was found between the severe TBI and control groups. There was an age at test effect, $\chi^2(1, N = 55) = 10.7$, $p = .001$, with older children being more likely to produce an accurate, complete, and abstract response.

Age-at-injury effects.   A significant difference was found between the young age at injury (<8 years) versus the older age at injury (>8 years) group on the ability to transform information, $\chi^2(1, N = 23)$, $p < .05$. As shown in Figure 2, children with earlier age at injury produced significantly fewer transformed propositions in their summaries as compared to children injured at later ages.

Linguistic and Cognitive Measures

A significant difference was found between the control group and the TBI group on the Formulated Sentences subtest of the CELF ($p = .01$). No group differences were identified on the other measures of the Block Design subtest of the WASI ($p = .13$), CVLT ($p = .28$), or the Vocabulary subtest of the WASI ($p = .07$). There was no significant gender effect between groups on discourse processing performance or on the other cognitive and linguistic measures.

As shown in Table 4, statistical analyses revealed a significant positive correlation between the discourse macrolevel score in transforming information in summary production and the Block Design subtest of the WASI ($r = .57$; $p = .02$). No significant correlations were found between this same discourse macrolevel measure and the other measures, including the memory measure, that is, CVLT ($r = -.17$; $p = .22$); the Vocabulary subtest (WASI; $r = .45$; $p = .07$); or the subtest of Sentence Formulation, that is, CELF ($r = .19$; $p = .18$).

DISCUSSION

Children with chronic stage (>2 years postinjury) and severe TBI had more difficulty transforming discourse information in the form of summaries. Our data indicated that children with severe TBI showed significantly less use of transformation macrorules in their summary productions as compared to control children. Instead, the summary texts of children with severe TBI contained predominantly untransformed information shown by copying or minimally paraphrasing the original content. Thus, the children with severe TBI were more likely to use a lower level "copy–delete" strategy in condensing information than typically developing children. Whereas the ability to transform information in summaries was significantly reduced in the severe TBI group, a limited number of these children were able to transform some information.

One caveat with using percentage of transformed t units is that this measure does not take into account differences in amount of t units produced. However, it is important to recognize that more t units are not necessarily better when producing transformed summaries. An individual can produce a concise high-level summary in just a few statements. We are currently investigating a complementary measure

TABLE 4
Spearman Rank Correlation Coefficients of Discourse Summary Score
With Other Cognitive and Linguistic Measures

Factor/Measure	r	p
WASI: Block Design	.57	.02*
CVLT: Monday List	−.17	.22
WASI: Vocabulary	.45	.07
CELF: Formulated Sentences	.19	.18

Note. WASI = Wechsler Abbreviated Scale of Intelligence Block Design raw score (Wechsler, 1999); CVLT = California Verbal Learning Test recall across Trials 1 through 5 of Monday List, raw score (Delis, Kramer, Kaplan, & Ober, 1986); WASI = Wechsler Abbreviated Scale of Intelligence Vocabulary raw score (Wechsler, 1999); CELF = Clinical Evaluation of Language Fundamentals Formulated Sentences raw score (Semel, Wiig, & Secord, 1995).

*$p < .05$.

of summary ability, namely a coherence and depth of processing rating, to characterize the qualitative aspect of the summary productions.

These results do not indicate that children with TBI form inaccurate mental representations of textual information. Rather, the summarization pattern shown by the majority of the children with severe TBI suggest that they continue to construct meaning at lower levels—being tied more to the lowest level of meaning as conveyed by the individual pieces of information. They displayed a marked reduction at intermediate levels of making inferences across sentences and at higher levels where summary statements are constructed to represent the global meaning of the text as a whole. It has been suggested that encoding information at lower–superficial levels makes the later retrieval of information more effortful and less likely since detail-based memory tends to be more transient over time (van Dijk, 1995). Moreover, the bias toward detail based encoding has been associated with low achievement in classroom contexts (Brown & Day, 1983; Johnson, 1983; Malone & Mastropieri, 1992; Stein & Kirby, 1992).

The study of summary performance extends previous discourse findings related to macrolevel processing in pediatric TBI (Chapman et al., 1992; Chapman, Levin, et al., 1995; Chapman et al., 1998; Chapman, Watkins, et al., 1997). In earlier studies, the study participants did not have specific instructions to focus on the main points. Rather, they were asked to retell the stories in as much detail as possible and their retells were subsequently analyzed according to whether or not the children included the important points. Using a more focused macrolevel discourse task that required selective reduction of information, children with severe TBI were found to perform significantly below their typically developing peers in developing higher level strategies of condensing information when tested 2 years or more after their brain injury.

Developmental studies reveal that the ability to transform information in summaries continues to evolve from a copy–delete strategy advancing to a more advanced strategy of transforming information at a more global level of semantic representation. This transition begins in early school years and is refined throughout adolescence and into college age (Brown, Day & Jones, 1983; Johnson, 1978). Most of the children in this study were injured prior to or during the stage when discourse transformation skills are emerging. Consequently, we postulate that the children who sustained severe TBI failed to develop later-emerging cognitive-linguistic skills required for summarization (Chapman & McKinnon, 2000). These data add to the mounting evidence that sustaining a brain injury in childhood prior to or during skill acquisition may alter or impede subsequent acquisition of that ability (Dennis, 2000; Ewing-Cobbs, Levin, Eisenberg, & Fletcher, 1987).

Furthermore, this study supports our hypothesis that a younger age at injury can have a more deleterious impact on the ability to acquire transformation rules. The children injured before 8 years of age performed lower than those injured after this age in transforming story information in their summary productions even though they all experienced similar levels of injury severity. In addition, even though the young age at injury (<8 years) group had a mean of 2 more years to recover from their injuries (injury test interval) than the older age at injury (>8 years) group, the young age at injury group performed significantly poorer. This pattern of poorer long-term outcome in children with younger age at injury is consistent with previous evidence of age at injury effects (Chapman et al., 1998; Levin, Song, Ewing-Cobbs, Chapman, & Mendelsohn, 2001).

Discourse macrolevel processing is related also to the status of particular cognitive skills such as memory and problem solving. Memory problems common to severe TBI may have contributed to difficulties in transforming information in their summaries. Summarization skills rely on the integrity of memory systems because the individual must comprehend the meaning, retrieve from short-term memory the most important information, and then transform the information through inferencing (Brown & Day, 1983; Chapman et al., 1999; Kinnunen & Vauras, 1995). However, performance on an episodic memory measure did not correlate with ability to transform discourse information in a summary in this study. That is, children with higher recall did not necessarily show an increased use of transformed information. In fact, if anything, the relation was the reverse of expected in that there was a negative correlation.

The failure to find a relation between episodic recall may not be surprising given the different processing demands of macrolevel text processing and detail-based recall of textual information. Conveying the global meaning of a discourse text in the form of a summary may be dissociated from the ability to recall specific details (Reyna & Brainerd, 1998). Empirical evidence has shown that individuals typically recall little of the explicit story information even on immediate recall (Kintsch & van Dijk, 1978). In efficient text processing, knowledge of the central meaning persists despite limited memory of the precise words and sentences. The negative relation between episodic memory and transformed discourse summaries (i.e., increased memory for specific words being associated with reduced use of transformed information) suggests that focusing on the explicit details may hamper an individual's ability to engage in macrolevel processing. Thus, focusing on the detail may occur at the expense of extracting a more generalized meaning. Moreover, this pattern may be exacerbated if the individual has cognitive limitations, although this possibility needs to be explored.

Problem-solving abilities may play a role in acquiring the ability to transform information as implicated by the significant correspondence between transformed information in summary productions and performance on the nonverbal problem-solving measure. Summarizing requires comprehension of the isolated facts that make up the whole discourse text, sorting them according to importance, and appreciating the relation of the isolated facts to the central meaning of the whole discourse text. Similarly, solving a block design puzzle involves breaking the whole into its parts and appreciating the relation of the parts to the whole. Previous discourse studies in brain-damaged populations have identified a significant relation between discourse macrolevel processing and cognitive performance on nonverbal problem-solving measures (Brookshire et al., 2000; Culhane, Chapman, & Levin, 1993).

The relation between the children's performance on the vocabulary subtest and the production of transformed summary information approached but failed to reach significance. Future studies should explore the nature of this relation. Previous studies have found a relation between vocabulary and discourse competence (Dennis & Lovett, 1990). Because summarizing information requires paraphrasing information at more generalized levels, a well-developed vocabulary may facilitate the expression of global ideas (Ulatowska & Chapman, 1994). In addition, the second structured measure of linguistic competence, that is, the ability to generate sentences from scrambled words, also did not correlate with the ability to produce transformed statements in the summary texts. This latter test probably taps a skill very different from that measured by sequencing ideas in connected language.

Whereas the cognitive measures used in this study revealed intriguing associations (problem solving–Block Design) and disparities (detail recall of word lists–CVLT) with discourse macrolevel measures, future studies should consider other cognitive measures to elucidate the cognitive mechanisms underlying discourse macrolevel processing. One important theoretical question is whether macrolevel processing in other cognitive domains, such as visual stimuli, is also impaired in pediatric brain injury. Second, whereas episodic memory for a list of words did not correspond to discourse macrolevel processing in this study, episodic memory as measured by tasks involving connected language may have been associated with discourse transformation ability. Moreover, measures of working memory capacity may be more informative and could be a key underlying cognitive prerequisite in supporting summarization skills. Summarization involves holding the information in working memory while mentally manipulating the information to make the necessary inferences to recode the content at a transformed level (van Dijk, 1995). Working memory limitations have a purported detrimental effect on inferential abilities (Worling, Humphries, & Tannock, 1999). In future research, it would be important to consider whether working memory capacity is a predictor of summarization skills in pediatric brain injury populations. In the linguistic domain, abstraction of similarities between two concepts could reveal higher level inferencing between two vocabulary items.

In addition to summarization, we evaluated discourse macrolevel processing on a task requiring formulation of the interpretive–generalized lesson expressed in a single statement. Whereas previous studies found significant impairments on generalized lesson responses in children with severe TBI at one year postinjury and longer (Chapman et al., 2001; Chapman, Watkins, et al., 1997), these results did not reveal a significant difference. Added to prior data showing that the ability to produce an interpretive statement recovers slower than recall of discourse informa-tion (Chapman et al., 2001), these findings suggest that summary ability may be even more vulnerable to the effects of severe TBI than constructing a single global statement.

One possible explanation for the failure to find a difference in this study may have been due to a ceiling effect. In the discourse stimuli used herein, the charac-ters were humans, whereas the characters in the previous studies were animals. To generate a lesson from the actions of animal characters requires another level of transposing the meaning from animal actions to human actions. Deciphering a les-son from human actions may be conceptually easier. However, the fact that there were age at test effects suggests that there is a developmental aspect implicating some degree of increasing complexity, even when humans are the actors from which the lesson has to be derived. Alternatively, the children may have had more exposure to the lesson that "money does not bring happiness." As a result of expe-rience, this lesson may have been more salient than those conveyed in previous dis-course stories. Additionally, the narrative stimuli used in earlier studies required more levels of inferencing to derive an interpretive statement, mitigating ceiling effects.

The inconsistency on the two discourse macrolevel tasks, that is, summary and lesson response, in children with severe TBI at least 2 years post injury is intrigu-ing. Why should a story lesson be less impaired after severe TBI than the ability to summarize and transform information? One possibility is that formulating a lesson relies more on real life experiences and less on manipulating large segments of tex-tual information. Alternatively, deriving lessons from narratives may be a more common learning experience whereas training in summarization skills is rarely provided (Hidi & Anderson, 1986). Summarization skills tend to be self-taught; however, children with learning problems have been shown to benefit from direct training, achieving higher levels of comprehension, memory, and improved sum-mary skills as reflected in transforming information (Kinnunen & Vauras, 1995).

One obvious question is whether or not the children with severe TBI understood what it means to give a summary. Perhaps differences between summary and les-son responses were due to the participant's understanding of the task. Both groups produced texts that were reduced in terms of the amount of language used to con-vey their summaries as compared to the original story. In fact, both groups showed a similar amount of reduction in the amount of language. Based on this finding, it was felt that the children with severe TBI did understand that they were to con-dense the original content. However, the severe TBI group differed from the con-trol group in the reduction strategies employed to produce summaries.

This study supports previous data suggesting that children who suffer severe TBI may show deficits on discourse macrolevel tasks (Chapman, Levin, et al., 1995; Chapman, Watkins, et al., 1997). The findings reported herein extend these findings to tasks that directly measure macrolevel processing, that is, summary tasks. Summarization requires cognitive manipulation of large chunks of information and inferencing across statements. Stein and Kirby (1992) have claimed that one can infer from an individual's summary the cognitive processes that went into its construction.

CONCLUSIONS AND IMPLICATIONS

Children who sustain a severe TBI prior to adolescence are at risk for failing to acquire the ability to transform information required for generating summaries. Moreover, children with earlier injuries may be at greater risk for long-term impairments in transforming information than children who are older at the time of injury. Future studies are needed to examine recovery of discourse macrolevel processing abilities in longitudinal studies.

Although our data do not bear directly on injury severity effects, some preliminary evidence indicates that children with milder levels of TBI severity are not as impaired as children with severe TBI (Chapman et al., 2001). Nonetheless, children with milder degrees of TBI may experience some reduced ability to engage in macrolevel processing (Chapman et al., 1992), but this requires further investigation.

Frontal brain regions have been implicated in tasks requiring organizing lengthy discourse information during retell (Chapman et al., 1992; Chapman et al., 2001) as well as on tasks requiring macrolevel processing (Nichelli et al., 1995). It would be of interest to evaluate whether a relation exists between discourse macrolevel processing and frontal lobe injury in children with TBI. It may be that site of lesion interacts with age at injury with frontal lesions showing an incremental impact on subsequent development of macrolevel strategies.

These results would suggest that constructing macrolevel texts in the form of summaries is more difficult than providing interpretive statements for children with severe TBI. We have previously argued that diagnostic and treatment protocols relating to information processing abilities should proceed from retells to interpretive statements, with the most difficult being summaries (Chapman et al., 1999). These results would support such a sequence.

For children with TBI, impaired macrolevel processing may contribute to poor school achievement. The ability to produce macrolevel texts is related to learning achievement in the classroom setting for typically developing children (Kinnunen & Vauras, 1995). It would be of interest to study whether discourse macrolevel processing is related to academic performance in children with TBI.

Summarization may prove to be a promising therapeutic milieu in pediatric TBI because a person's ability to produce a summary directly represents how well he or she comprehends, remembers, and is able to use this information for later learning. The ability to summarize relies not only on linguistic competence, but also on cognitive processes, and is correlated with academic achievement (Brown & Day, 1983). The evidence that learning skills in low achievers can be enhanced has stimulated interest in macrolevel processing in TBI (Kinnunen & Vauras, 1995; Stein & Kirby, 1992). Students' success in school relies largely on their repertoire of learning strategies and metacognitive skills (Brown & Day, 1983).

If children with TBI have greater than expected difficulties in producing macrolevel texts, then perhaps more appropriate interventions could be designed to give them explicit training in macrolevel strategies, that is, "when" and "how" to apply metacognitive knowledge to utilize macrolevel processing. Because earlier age at injury has an increased detrimental effect on discourse processing, perhaps earlier interventions could help to mitigate these age effects. Future clinical trials that incorporate summary training versus more traditional approaches would be beneficial in developing more appropriate treatments with the hope of enhancing learning achievement in children with TBI.

ACKNOWLEDGMENTS

This work was supported by the National Institute of Neurological Disorders and Stroke (Grant 2RO1 NS 21889–16).

We gratefully acknowledge the contributions of Kim Davies and Steve Roach of the Children's Medical Center in Dallas, TX; Becky Yates and Frank McDonald from Our Children's House at Baylor University Medical Center in Dallas, TX; and Jacquelyn Gamino for her assistance with editing the final manuscript. We also sincerely thank all the children and families whose commitment made this project possible.

REFERENCES,

Brookshire, B. L., Chapman, S. B., Song, J., & Levin, H. S. (2000). Cognitive and linguistic correlates of children's discourse after closed head injury: A three year follow-up. *Journal of the International Neuropsychological Society, 6,* 741–751.

Brown, A. L., & Day, J. D. (1983). Macrorules for summarizing texts: The development of expertise. *Journal of Verbal Learning and Verbal Behavior, 22,* 1–14.

Brown, A. L., Day, J. D., & Jones, R. S. (1983). The development of plans for summarizing texts. *Child Development, 54,* 968–979.

Chadwick, O., Rutter, M., Brown, G., Shaffer, D., & Traub, M. A. (1981). A prospective study of children with head injuries. II. Cognitive sequela. *Psychological Medicine, 11,* 49–61.

Chapman, S. B., Culhane, K. A., Levin, H. S., Harward, H., Mendelsohn, D., Ewing-Cobbs, L., Fletcher, J. M., & Bruce, D. (1992). Narrative discourse after closed head injury in children and adolescents. *Brain and Language, 43,* 42–65.

Chapman, S. B., Levin, H. S., & Lawyer, S. L. (1999). Communication problems resulting from brain injury in children: Special issues of assessment and management. In S. McDonald, L. Togher, & C.

Code (Eds.), *Brain damage, behavior, and cognitive series*. Hove, East Sussex, UK: Lawrence Erlbaum Associates, Inc.

Chapman, S. B., Levin, H. S., Matejka, J., Harward, H. N., & Kufera, J. (1995). Discourse ability in head injured children: Consideration of linguistic, psychosocial & cognitive factors. *Journal of Head Trauma Rehabilitation, 10,* 36–54.

Chapman, S. B., Levin, H. S., Wanek, A., Weyrauch, J., & Kufera, J. (1998). Discourse after closed head injury in young children. *Brain and Language, 61,* 420–449.

Chapman, S. B., & McKinnon, L. (2000). Discussion of developmental plasticity: Factors affecting cognitive outcome after pediatric traumatic brain injury. *Journal of Communication Disorders, 33,* 333–344.

Chapman, S. B., McKinnon, L., Levin, H. S., Song, J., Meier, M. C., & Chiu, S. (2001). *Longitudinal outcome of verbal discourse in children with traumatic brain injury: Three-year follow-up.* Journal of Head Trauma Rehabilitation, *16*(5), 1–15.

Chapman, S. B., Ulatowska, H. K., Franklin, L. R., Shobe, A. E., Thompson, J. L., & McIntire, D. D. (1997). *Proverb interpretation in fluent aphasia and Alzheimer's disease: Implications beyond abstract thinking.* Aphasiology, *11,* 337–350.

Chapman, S. B., Ulatowska, H. K., King, K., Johnson, J. K., & McIntire, D. D. (1995). Discourse in early Alzheimer's disease versus normal advanced aging. *American Journal of Speech-Language Pathology, 4*(4), 124–129.

Chapman, S. B., Watkins, R., Gustafson, C., Moore, S., Levin, H. S., & Kufera, J. A. (1997). Narrative discourse in children with closed head injury, children with language impairment, and typically developing children. *American Journal of Speech-Language Pathology, 6*(2), 66–76.

Chapman, S. B., Zientz, J., Weiner, M., Rosenburg, R., Frawley, W., & Burns, M. H. (in press). Discourse changes in early Alzheimer's disease, mild cognitive impairment, and normal aging. *Journal of Alzheimer's Disease and Associated Disorders.*

Culhane, K. A., Chapman, S. B., & Levin, H.S. (1993, February). *The relationship of discourse and cognitive task performance following closed head injury.* Paper presented at the International Neuropsychological Society Meeting, San Antonio, TX.

Delis, D. C., Kramer, J., & Kaplan, E. (1984). *The California Proverb Test.* Unpublished protocol.

Delis, D. C., Kramer, J. H., Kaplan, E., & Ober, B. A. (1986). *The California Verbal Learning Test: Research edition.* New York: The Psychological Corporation.

Dennis, M. (2000). Developmental plasticity in children: the role of biological risk, development, time, and reserve, *Journal of Communication Disorders, 33,* 321–332.

Dennis, M., Barnes, M. A., Donnelly, R. E., Wilkinson, M., & Humphreys, R. P. (1996). Appraising and managing knowledge: Metacognitive skills after childhood head injury. *Developmental Neuropsychology, 12,* 77–103.

Dennis, M., Barnes, M. A., Wilkinson, M., & Humphreys, R. P. (1998). How children with head injury represent real and deceptive emotion in short narratives. *Brain and Language, 61,* 450–483.

Dennis, M., Guger, S., Roncadin, C., Barnes, M., & Schachar, R. (2001). Attentional-inhibitory control and social behavioral regulation after childhood closed head injury: Do biological, developmental, and recovery variables predict outcome? *Journal of the International Neuropsychological Society, 7,* 683–692.

Dennis, M., & Lovett, M. W. (1990). Discourse ability in children after brain damage. In Y. Joanette & H. H. Brownell (Eds.), *Discourse ability and brain damage: Theoretical and empirical perspectives.* New York: Springer-Verlag.

Dennis, M., Purvis, K., Barnes, M. A., Wilkinson, M., & Winner, E. (2001). Understanding of literal truth, ironic criticism, and deceptive praise following childhood head injury. *Brain and Language, 78,* 1–16.

Ewing-Cobbs, L., Levin, H. S., Eisenberg, H. M., & Fletcher, J. M. (1987). Language functions following closed-head injury in children and adolescents. *Journal of Clinical and Experimental Neuropsychology, 9,* 575–592.

Hidi, S., & Anderson, V. (1986). Producing written summaries: Task demands, cognitive, operations, and implications for instruction. *Review of Educational Research, 56,* 473–493.

Hunt, K. W. (1965). *Grammatical structures written at three grade levels.* Research Report No. 3, Champaign, IL: National Council of Teachers of English.

Jennett, B., & Bond, M. (1975). Assessment of outcome after severe brain damage. *Lancet, 1,* 480–484.

Johnson, N. S. (1978). *A structural analysis of the development of story recall and summarization.* Unpublished doctoral thesis, University of California, San Diego.

Johnson, N. S. (1983). What do you do if you can tell the whole story? The development of summarization skills. In K. E. Nelson (Ed.), *Children's Language* (pp. 315–383). New York: Gardner.

Kinnunen, R., & Vauras, M. (1995). Comprehension monitoring and the level of comprehension in high- and low-achieving primary school children's reading. *Learning and Instruction, 5,* 143–165.

Kintsch, W., & van Dijk, T. (1978). Toward a model of text comprehension and production. *Psychological Review, 85,* 363–394.

Kirby, J. R. (1988). Style, strategy, and skill in reading. In R. R. Schmeck (Ed.), *Learning strategies and learning styles* (pp. 229–274). New York: Plenum.

Kirby, J. R., & Cantwell, R. H. (1985). Use of advance organizers to facilitate higher-level text comprehension. *Human Learning, 4,* 159–168.

Kirby, J. R., & Pedwell, D. (1991). Students' approaches to summarization. *Educational Psychology, 11,* 297–307.

Kirby, J. R., & Probert, P. J. (1988, September). *Instruction in the processes of summarization.* Paper presented to the International Congress of Psychology, Sydney, Australia.

Levin, H. S., & Eisenberg, H. M. (1979). Neuropsychological impairment after closed head injury in children and adolescents. *Journal of Pediatric Psychology, 4,* 389–402.

Levin, H. S., Ewing-Cobbs, L., & Eisenberg, H. (1995).Neurobehavioral outcome of pediatric closed head injury. In S. H. Broman & M. E. Michel (Eds.), *Traumatic head injury in children* (pp. 70–94). New York: Oxford.

Levin, H. S., Song, J., Ewing-Cobbs, L., Chapman, S. B., & Mendelsohn, D. (2001). Word fluency in relation to severity of closed head injury, associated frontal brain lesions, and age at injury in children. *Neuropsychologia, 39,* 122–131.

Liang, K. Y., & Zeger, S. L. (1986). Longitudinal data analysis using a generalized linear model. *Biometrika, 73,* 13–22.

Malone, L. D., & Mastropieri, M. A. (1992). Reading comprehension instruction: Summarization and self-monitoring training for students with learning disabilities. *Exceptional Children, 58,* 270–279.

Nichelli, P., Grafman, J., Pietrini, P., Clark, K., Lee, K. Y., & Miletich, R. (1995). Where the brain appreciates the moral of a story. *Neuroreport, 6,* 2309–2313.

Revelle, G. L., Wellman, H. M., & Karabenick, J. D. (1985). Comprehension monitoring in preschool children. *Child Development, 56,* 654–663.

Reyna, R., & Brainerd, C. J. (1998). Fuzzy-trace theory and false memory: New frontiers. *Journal of Experimental Child Psychology, 71,* 194–209.

Semel, E., Wiig, E. H., & Secord, W. A. (1995). *Clinical evaluation of language fundamentals* (3rd ed.). San Antonio: Psychological.

Stein, B. L., & Kirby, J. R. (1992). The effects of text absent and text present conditions on summarization and recall of text. *Journal of Reading Behavior, 24,* 217–232.

Teasdale, G., & Jennett, B. (1974). Assessment of coma and impaired consciousness: A practical scale. *Lancet, 13*(2), 81–84.

Ulatowska, H. K., & Chapman, S. B. (1994). Discourse microstructure in aphasia. In R. L. Bloom, L. K. Obler, S. DeSanti, & J. S. Ehrlich (Eds.), *Discourse analysis and applications* (pp. 29–46). Hillsdale, NJ: Lawrence Erlbaum Associates, Inc.

van Dijk, T. A. (1995). On macrostructure, mental models, and other inventions: A brief personal his-
tory of the Kintsch-van Dijk Theory. In C. A. Weaver, S. Mannes, & C. R. Fletcher (Eds.), *Discourse comprehension* (pp. 383–410). Hillsdale, NJ: Lawrence Erlbaum Associates, Inc.

Vauras, M., Kinnunen, R., & Kuusela, L. (1994). Development of text processing skills in high-, aver-
age-, and low-achieving primary school children. *Journal of Reading Behavior, 26,* 361–389.

Wechsler, D. (1999). *Wechsler Abbreviated Scale of Intelligence.* San Antonio, TX: Psychological.

Worling, D. E., Humphries, T., & Tannock, R. (1999). Spatial and emotional aspects of language
inferencing in nonverbal learning disabilities. *Brain and Language, 70,* 220–239.

Yorkston, K. J., Jaffee, K. M., Liao, S., & Polissar, N. L. (1999). Recovery of written language production in children with traumatic brain injury: Outcomes at one year. *Aphasiology, 13,* 691–700.

Yorkston, K. M., Jaffe, K. M., Polissar, N. L., Liao, S., & Fay, G. C. (1997). Written language produc-
tion and neuropsychological function in children with traumatic brain injury. *Archives of Physical Medicine and Rehabilitation, 78,* 1096–1002.

APPENDIX A
Narrative Overview and Original Stimulus of "The Rich Man and the Shoemaker"

Overview

"The Rich Man and the Shoemaker" introduces the main characters as a poor but happy shoemaker and his rich, unhappy neighbor who cannot sleep due to the constant worrying about his money and the shoemaker's singing. The first episode ends with the rich man giving the shoemaker one hundred pounds of money as a plan to keep him from singing happy songs. The second episode is considered a turning point in which the previous events have led to a role reversal for the two characters. Now it is the shoemaker who has become restless, worrisome, and unhappy. The shoemaker's wife advises the shoemaker to give the money back to the rich man because she prefers to be poor and to hear him sing than to be rich. The shoemaker promptly returns the money to the rich man and exclaims, "I want my life back." Therefore, to realize the gist of the story, one has to appreciate the role reversal situation for the two main characters. Specifically, this story revolves around the generalized lesson that money is not the root of happiness.

Stimulus

Episode 1.   There was once a poor shoemaker who worked very hard to make the money his family needed. Even though he was poor, he was happy and always sang as he worked. The people of the village would come to listen to his happy songs. Next door to the shoemaker lived a rich man. He had all the things he wanted, but still he was not happy. All he could do was worry about his money. He was so scared that someone would take his money that he could not sleep most nights. Then when he would finally fall asleep, the shoemaker's singing would wake him up. The same thing happened every night and every morning. The rich man began to get more and more upset about the happy songs of the shoemaker. The rich man began to think of a way to make the shoemaker stop singing. One morning the rich man knocked at the shoemaker's door. The shoemaker was so surprised to see the rich man because he obviously would not need to have his shoes fixed. Indeed the rich man had not come to see about his shoes. He wanted to talk to the shoemaker about money. The rich man said to the shoemaker, "You are the happiest man I have ever known. Here! I have a surprise for you. You have earned it with all your happy songs." He gave the shoemaker a heavy bag of money. Then the rich man walked home, thinking to himself that he would finally get some sleep.

Episode 2.   The shoemaker excitedly ran into his house to count the money. "One hundred pounds!" he said in surprise. "This is enough money for us to live on for the rest of our lives if we spend it wisely. I must not tell anyone, not even my wife." Now all the shoemaker could do was worry about his money. He did not sing anymore. He just thought of hiding places for his money. First, he hid it under the bed; then under the bed covers. He was scared that his wife would find the money when she went to bed. So he took the bag outside and hid it in the chicken house in the yard. While the shoemaker looked for places to hide his money, the rich man slept. It was now the shoemaker who had a sleepless night, tossing and turning. The shoemaker thought he would sleep once he found a good hiding place for the money, but no place seemed safe enough. Finally one day the shoemaker's wife said, "What is wrong? I have never seen you so unhappy. Please tell me what the matter is." The shoemaker took the money bag from the chicken house and told his wife they were rich. "I should be happy, but I'm not. I have never known such worry." His wife told him to take the money back to the rich man. "It's not so bad to be poor. I would rather hear you sing than have money." The excited shoemaker took the bag of money and ran to his neighbor. His knock woke the rich man. "I'm sorry, but I cannot keep your one hundred pounds," the shoemaker said. "I want my life back."

Examples of Transformed and Untransformed Narratives and Lessons (T = transformed, UT = untransformed, I = incorrect)

Sample A: Male child with severe TBI secondary to a motor vehicle collision. Age at injury 5.7 years. Age at test 12.6 years. Glasgow Outcome Scale: moderate recovery

Summary:
The shoemaker was um, was poor (UT) / yet he was very happy (UT) / and he always sang songs and everything (UT) / And the rich man was worried 'cause he had to keep track of his money (UT) / and he was always, didn't like hearing his singing (UT) / So he gave him some money (UT) / and then the shoemaker was all worried (UT) / and he hid the money under the bed (UT) / and then he hid the money under the bed covers (UT) / and then he hid the money in the chicken house (UT) / And his wife finally made him give the money back. (UT) /

Lesson: Don't steal anyone's money. (I)

Observations:
The child showed good reduction of information, however, failed to transform any of the information (0% transformation). Notice the child's use of correct, important information. However, the child produced specific detail qualities from the story which were closely paraphrased from the story. Therefore, the child did not demonstrate a clear understanding of the deeper meaning of the story in the summary or in the lesson statement.

Sample B: Male child. Age at test 12.9 years (Age-equivalent control)

Summary:
There's a shoemaker who is really, really happy about his life (T) / and there is a rich man who doesn't like his life and who keeps on worrying about his money (T) / Well, finally, the rich man gives the shoemaker a lot of money, switching places in life with him (T) / And then the poor man learns his lesson about taking the money and thinks, "I should have left my happy life alone." (T) /

Lesson: Money can't make you happy. (T)

Observations:
Notice that the child condensed and transformed the information into his own words (100% transformation), using relatively long sentences with clausal embeddings. With regard to the information, the child produced coherent, correctly ordered ideas that revolved around the role reversal for the characters, thus revealing the central meaning. Additionally, the child clearly stated the meaning of the story using a shortened lesson statement.

DEVELOPMENTAL NEUROPSYCHOLOGY, 25(1&2), 61–83

Components of Executive Function in Typically Developing and Head-Injured Children

Bonnie Brookshire
Private Practice
Houston, TX

Harvey S. Levin
Cognitive Neuroscience Laboratory
Departments of Physical Medicine and Rehabilitation,
Neurosurgery, and Psychiatry and Behavioral Sciences
Baylor College of Medicine
Houston, TX

James X. Song
Department of Biometry
Bayer Pharmaceuticals
West Haven, CT

Lifang Zhang
Cognitive Neuroscience Laboratory
Departments of Physical Medicine and Rehabilitation
Houston, TX

To identify the key components of executive functions (EFs) in children following traumatic brain injury (TBI), data from a series of EF tests administered to 286 pediatric TBI patients at least 3 years postinjury were subjected to an exploratory factor analysis. A 5-factor model included discourse, EFs (e.g., problem solving, planning), processing speed (e.g., coding), declarative memory, and motor speed. Confirmatory

Requests for reprints should be sent to Harvey S. Levin, Cognitive Neuroscience Laboratory, Baylor College of Medicine, 6560 Fannin Street, Ste. 1144, Houston, TX 77030. E-mail: hlevin@bcm.tmc.edu factor analysis based on data obtained from 265 pediatric TBI patients at 3 months postinjury disclosed that the 5-factor model provided a good fit to the data. A second exploratory analysis of the 3-month postinjury data disclosed a 4-factor model in which processing speed and motor speed measures loaded on a common factor. Severity of TBI and age at test had significant effects on all factors in both the 5- and 4-factor models. Adaptive functioning, as measured by the Vineland Adaptive Behavioral Scale–Revised, was moderately related to factor scores at 3 years or longer postinjury, but weakly related to factor scores obtained at 3 months postinjury. The factor scores could be used in clinical trials to facilitate data reduction and appear to have validity as indicators of TBI outcome.

"Executive" implies control of cognitive processes (Miller, 2000), and has been invoked to describe functions that are supervisory (Shallice & Burgess, 1991), managerial (Grafman & Litvan, 1999), and goal directed (Duncan, 1986). Cognitive theorists have proposed that executive functions (EFs) include (a) maintenance of a problem solving set for future goals (Pennington, Bennetto, McAleer, & Roberts, 1996), (b) organization of behavior over time (Denckla, 1996), (c) flexibility in problem solving, (d) self-monitoring and self-regulation (Borkowski & Burke, 1996), (e) conforming to rules of social behavior (Price, Daffner, Stowe, & Mesulam, 1990), (f) skillful use of strategies (Graham & Harris, 1996), and (g) utilizing reward and punishment to facilitate learning (Giedd et al., 1996). From a neuroscience perspective, we view EFs as the capacity to maintain goals and the means to achieve them while resisting interference (Miller & Cohen, 2001). According to this view, frontally guided, distributed networks mediate top-down control of behavior. Executive functions, which involve both monitoring and control of behavior, interact with declarative memory and processing speed but are distinct abilities.

However, no classification of EFs is universally accepted, there is no consensus on the essential EFs or their most efficient measures, and the key dimensions common to frequently cited EFs in children have not been identified. Identification of the dimensions underlying EFs will facilitate the development of appropriate test batteries to investigate relations between specific EFs and pathophysiological indexes of TBI, facilitate design of effective outcome protocols for clinical trials, and assist in the development of cognitive probes for use in research and clinical studies of functional magnetic resonance imaging (fMRI). Consequently, the goals of this study were to identify the key factors of EFs in relation to other cognitive abilities, elucidate the relation of the factor scores to injury variables, and analyze the relation of EF factor scores to well-established measures of adaptive functioning.

Neuroscience research using infrahuman primate models (Goldman, 1974), functional brain imaging (Cabeza & Nyberg, 2000; Casey et al., 1997), and studies of patients with focal brain lesions (Eslinger, Grattan, Damasio, & Damasio, 1992; Marlowe, 1992) have indicated that EFs depend on the integrity of prefrontal cortex and its circuity (Anderson, Levin, & Jacobs, 2002; Giedd et al., 1996; Luciana & Nelson, 1998), which comprise a widely distributed neural network with a relatively late maturational trajectory (Diamond, 1991; Huttenlocher & Dabholkar, 1997). This neuroanatomic organization of EFs is vulnerable to nonmissile traumatic brain injury (TBI), which frequently produces prefrontal lesions and disconnects this region from associated cortical and subcortical areas (Adams, Graham, Scott, Parker, & Doyle, 1980; Levin et al., 1997). Despite recovery by most children sustaining severe and moderate TBI to the normal range on traditional tests of intellectual and language functions (Levin, Eisenberg, Wigg, & Kobayashi, 1982; Levin, Fletcher, Kusnerik, et al., 1996), we have found that EF deficits persist on measures of problem solving, planning, response modulation (Levin, Culhane, et al., 1994; Levin, Mendelsohn, et al., 1994; Levin, Song, Ewing-Cobbs, & Roberson, 2001), and production of oral and written narratives (Chapman et al., 1992; Dennis, Barnes, Wilkinson, & Humphreys, 1998; Dennis & Lovett, 1990).

The factor structure of EF tasks has been explored in one study of children following TBI. Levin, Fletcher, Kufera, et al. (1996) examined the factor structure of EF measures in a group of head-injured and normal children by completing a principal components analysis of data collected from a series of tests designed to measure concept formation and problem solving, planning, verbal fluency, design fluency, memory, and response modulation. The five-factor solution obtained in this initial study included the following: Conceptual-Productivity (e.g., word fluency), Planning (e.g., Tower of London), Schema (e.g., Twenty Questions Test), Semantic Clustering (e.g., California Verbal Learning Test), and Inhibition (e.g., Go-No Go task). Severity of injury had a significant effect on four factors and age at testing had a significant effect for three of the five factors. In view of the relatively small sample size of this initial factor analytic study, Levin, Fletcher, Kufera, et al. (1996) recommended further research to explore the dimensionality of the EF measures with a larger sample of head-injured children, using alternative methods of factor analysis.

This study expands the Levin, Fletcher, Kufera, et al. (1996) article, using both exploratory and confirmatory factor analytic methods on measures of executive functioning and other cognitive abilities and assessing a larger group of typically developing and head-injured children. Goals of this study were (a) replication of the previous factor analytic findings in a much larger sample of TBI children at early or late stages of recovery, including a larger number of EF test variables to increase the reliability of the factors; (b) determination of the relation of the obtained factors to severity of injury; and (c) elucidation of the relation of factor scores to more ecologically valid measures of adaptive functioning.

From a theoretical perspective, we view EFs as the capacity to maintain goals and the means to achieve them while resisting interference (Miller & Cohen, 2001). According to this view, frontally guided, distributed networks mediate top-down control of behavior. Executive functions, which involve both monitoring and control of behavior, interact with declarative memory and processing speed, but are distinct abilities.

METHOD

Participants

Three hundred ninety children, including 104 typically developing children and 286 head-injured patients (62 mild, 90 moderate, and 134 severe), were included in the initial analyses based on the following selection criteria: (a) age 5 to 18 years at the time of testing; and (b) hospitalization for nonpenetrating head trauma due to sudden acceleration or deceleration of the freely moving head or being struck with a blunt object. Exclusion criteria included the following: (a) injury due to child abuse; (b) a history of substance abuse, mental retardation, or learning disability; (c) previous head injury resulting in hospitalization; and (d) preinjury history of diagnosed neurologic or psychiatric disorder. The head-injured patients had been recruited from consecutive admissions to Texas hospitals in Houston, Dallas, and Galveston. Severity of injury was determined according to the lowest postresuscitation Glasgow Coma Scale (GCS; Teasdale & Jennett, 1974) score (3–8 = severe, 9–12 = moderate, and 13–15 = mild). In addition to the GCS score, computed tomography (CT) within 24 hr after injury and magnetic resonance imaging (MRI) performed at least 3 months postinjury showed no evidence of a brain lesion for an injury to be classified as mild. Children with imaging evidence of a brain lesion and a GCS score of 13–15 were classified as sustaining a moderate TBI. The sample of 286 patients for the exploratory factor analysis (Table 1) included 171 children who were recruited during their initial hospitalization (prospective cohort) and serially tested up to 36 months postinjury (only data for 36 months were used in the analysis for the prospective cohort) and 115 patients recruited from a retrospective cohort who were tested only once at least 36 months postinjury. Head-injured children in both cohorts were selected from the same hospital populations without regard to their outcome, provided that they were conscious survivors and capable of participating in neuropsychological testing. We combined the two cohorts in this analysis to obtain a larger sample, as they had similar performances in our previous studies (Levin et al., 1993). Typically developing children were recruited from the Dallas community to provide a comparison group and were tested on one occasion. Our previous studies have dis-

TABLE 1
Demographic and Clinical Features of TBI Groups Assessed at Least 36
Months Postinjury and Typically Developing Control Participants

Variable	Control[a] M	SD	Mild[b] M	SD	Moderate[c] M	SD	Severe[d] M	SD
Age at injury (years)	—		7.4	3.8	8.1	3.6	7.6	3.7
Age at test (years)	10.4_{abc}	3.2	11.7_a	3.6	12.4_b	3.2	12.4_c	3.6
Postinjury interval (years)	—		4.3	1.8	4.3	1.9	4.8	2.5
GCS score	—		14.5_a	0.9	12.6_a	2.1	5.6_a	1.7
Gender (percent)								
Male	61		69		61		62	
Female	39		31		39		38	
Parental education (years)	14.1_a	2.5	15.2_{ab}	2.8	13.6_b	2.9	13.3_{ab}	2.7

Note.   Common columns subscripts denote significant (≤ 0.05) pairwise contrasts of mean scores. TBI = traumatic brain injury; GCS = Glasgow Coma Scale (Teasdale & Jennett, 1974).
[a]$n = 104$. [b]$n = 62$. [c]$n = 90$. [d]$n = 134$.

closed no consistent differences in cognitive performance among samples of children tested at these different sites in Texas.

Demographic and clinical features of the comparison and head-injured groups are presented in Table 1. Mean age at injury and mean interval since injury did not differ significantly among the head-injured groups. However, mean age at test of the typically developing children, 10.4 years, was significantly younger than the three head-injured groups. Approximately 60% of each group were male. Although the groups differed significantly in parental education, average educational level was at least high school. The data of typically developing children were used along with the data of 286 head-injured patients to generate the intercorrelation matrix and to identify the 20 variables with the strongest correlations.

To examine the factor structure of EF measures in children who had a relatively brief injury–test interval, 265 head-injured patients (73 mild, 94 moderate, and 98 severe) in the prospective cohort who completed 3-month evaluations were included in the analyses, using the aforementioned selection and exclusion criteria (see Table 2). Mean age at injury of these severity groups was similar, as was their mean interval since injury. Severity groups were comparable in gender and parental education.

Materials and Procedure

Table 3 summarizes the procedures included in a battery designed to assess EFs in typically developing and head-injured children. This battery had been admin-

TABLE 2
Demographic and Clinical Features of TBI Patients Assessed at
3 Months Postinjury

| Variable | TBI Patients | | | | | |
| | Mild[a] | | Moderate[b] | | Severe[c] | |
	M	SD	M	SD	M	SD
Age at injury (years)	9.7	3.2	10.3	3.1	10.1	3.3
At at test (years)	10.0	3.2	10.6	3.1	10.4	3.3
Postinjury interval (years)	0.3	0.07	0.3	0.06	0.3	0.08
GCS score	14.6$_a$	0.67	12.3$_a$	2.1	5.7$_a$	1.8
Gender (percent)						
Male	58		54		58	
Female	43		46		42	
Parental education (years)	14.3$_a$	2.5	13.2$_a$	3.0	13.6	2.5

Note.   Across columns, the subscript denotes significant (≤ 0.05) pairwise contrasts. TBI = traumatic brain injury; GCS = Glasgow Coma Scale (Teasdale & Jennett, 1974).
    [a]$n = 73$. [b]$n = 94$. [c]$n = 98$.

istered to TBI patients at least 36 months postinjury (retrospective cohort) participating in a cross-sectional study and to TBI patients (prospective cohort) in a longitudinal study who were tested at 3 and 36 months postinjury. As reviewed in the Introduction, our conceptualization of EFs included flexibility in problem solving, planning, self-regulation, skillful use of strategies, and metacognition, which interact with other cognitive abilities such as long-term memory and processing speed. Although this battery included domains such as processing speed and declarative memory, we were interested in identifying EF factors in the context of other cognitive abilities. Examiners coded the EF procedures and other tests for validity immediately after completing testing. To mitigate variability due to failure to understand the instructions or lack of cooperation, data for each patient were screened and analysis was limited to those measures that the examiner had administered according to standard procedure or with slight modification (e.g., use of nonpreferred hand due to a cast on the patient's preferred upper extremity). However, if a child was unable to provide valid data for a test, it did not affect inclusion of the patient's valid data on other measures. Consequently, the sample size varied slightly across various tests. Each of the EF procedures generated one or more measures. Based on an intercorrelation matrix, 20 measures that obtained the highest correlations were selected for exploratory factor analysis. With the exception of the Peabody Picture Vocabulary Test–Revised (PPVT–R) standard score, raw scores were analyzed for all of the measures.

TABLE 3

Measures Included in a Battery Designed to Assess Executive Functioning in Typically Developing Children and TBI Patients

Domain	Procedure	Description	Measures
Problem solving and planning	Porteus Mazes (Porteus, 1965)	A series of mazes of increasing difficulty	Number correctly completed—number attempted*
	Wisconsin Card Sorting Test (Grant & Berg, 1948; Heaton, Chelune, Talley, Kay, & Curtis, 1993)	Sort cards according to relevant dimensions	Percentage of conceptual responses.* Number of categories
	Tower of London (Shallice, 1982)	Plan and execute a series of moves to rearrange colored beads on rods to match a model	Percentage solved in three trials.* Planning time
	Twenty Questions Test (Denney & Denney, 1973)	Identify a target picture by asking as few questions as possible	Percentage of hypothesis questions. Percentage of constraint questions*
Resource allocation	Divided Attention (Hiscock, Kinsbourne, Samuels, & Krause, 1987)	Child completes finger-tapping task with and without distraction (saying a nursery rhyme)	Difference in score between single task and divided attention condition expressed as a ratio*
Productivity	Verbal Fluency (Benton, 1968)	Generate words beginning with a specific letter in 60 sec	Total number of words summed over three letters*
	Design fluency (Jones-Gotman & Milner, 1977)	Draw abstract designs in 3 min (free condition); designs must contain four lines (fixed condition)	Number of designs drawn under free and fixed* conditions
Processing speed	Semantic Memory Verification Speed (Baddeley & Wilson, 1988)	Judge the veracity of 16 aurally presented statements (e.g., "Cats can fly," "Bicycles have wheels")	Accuracy and latency* of judgments
	WISC–R Coding (Wechsler, 1974)	Rapid graphomotor production of forms corresponding to specific numbers	Number of forms correctly produced in 2 min*

(continued)

TABLE 3 (Continued)

Domain	Procedure	Description	Measures
Motor functioning and response inhibition	Go–No Go Task (Drewe, 1975)	Child presses a key on "go" trials and withholds response on "no-go" trials in response to stimuli presented in this computer task	Total number of correct and false positive responses, ratio of false positive to total number of responses. Mean reaction time*
	Motor Sequencing (Luria, 1966)	Child imitates a sequence of unilateral hand movements	Total number of sequencing errors; total time required to complete sequences*
	Conflictual Motor Responses (Luria, 1966)	Child is instructed to perform a conflictual motor task in response to examiner's motor response (i.e., examiner taps once and child taps twice)	Total number of error responses in conflictual and nonconflictual conditions
	Grooved Pegboard (Matthews & Kløve, 1964)	Child places pegs into angled slotted holes	Time to complete task*
Memory	California Verbal Learning Test (Delis, Kramer, Kaplan, & Ober, 1986)	Five recall trials of 15 words belonging to three semantic categories	Total number of words recalled*; percentage of words clustered according to semantic category*
	Metamemory	Questions about what conditions facilitate memory	Score* based on number of conditions mentioned

Language and Discourse		
Peabody Picture Vocabulary Test (Dunn & Dunn, 1981)	Child is requested to select one of four pictures that corresponds best to a spoken word	Standard score based on total number of words correctly identified*
Rapid Automatized Naming (Denckla & Rudel, 1974)	Child rapidly names pictures of five common objects reproduced 10 times in a 5 × 10 array	Time required to complete the task*; errors and hesitancies
Discourse measures (Chapman et al., 1992)		
Episodes	Story components (i.e., setting, action, and resolution) that form an episode	Percentage of episodic structures (number of components in child's story divided by the number in the original story)*
Core propositions	Core information units in the child's story	Number of units in child's story divided by the number of units in the original story*
Gist propositions	Propositions in the child's story that contain essential meaning	Number of propositions in child's story divided by the number of propositions in the original story*

Note. Test variables selected for inclusion in factor analysis are denoted by an asterisk. TBI = traumatic brain injury. WISC–R = Wechsler Intelligence Scale for Children–Revised.

RESULTS

Exploratory Factor Analysis of the Outcome Data Obtained From Typically Developing and Head-Injured Children Who Were at Least 36 Months Postinjury

Exploratory Factor Analysis was performed on the 20 measures marked with an asterisk in Table 3. The data were obtained from the typically developing children, TBI patients in the retrospective cohort, and the 36-month follow-up examinations of the prospective study patients to ensure that the analysis reflected long-term outcome. The common variance (communality) in each variable was extracted and the squared multiple correlations were used as prior communality estimates. With oblique rotation, the rotated factor pattern was reviewed. Consequently, covariation, rather than total variance of the data set, was used to identify a five-factor model that appeared to identify separable dimensions representing shared variability (54% of total variance), thus providing the best resolution of simple structure. Significant factor loading was defined as a loading of at least 0.4. The Kaiser-Meyer-Olkin Measure of Sampling Adequacy was 0.90 reflecting good partial correlations between each pair of variables after controlling for all other variables.

As reflected by the factor loadings presented in Table 4, Factor 1 (Discourse) is defined by discourse measures of essential information and organization as well as the PPVT–R measure of oral receptive vocabulary. Factor 2 (Problem Solving) is defined by multiple measures considered to assess planning, problem solving, productivity, working memory, and metamemory. Measures associated with planning and problem solving include percentage of conceptual responses obtained on the Wisconsin Card Sorting Test, number of mazes completed in relation to the number attempted on the Porteus Mazes, and percentage of problems solved in three trials on the Tower of London. Problem solving and productivity are associated with the number of words and designs produced on the verbal and design fluency tests, and allocation of resources in the divided attention task, as reflected by finger tapping performance in the single task relative to the dual task condition. Adequate responses to "how to remember" questions were used to measure metamemory ability. Measures loading on Factor 3 (Processing Speed) include the Coding raw score from the Wechsler Intelligence Scale for Children–Revised (WISC–R), speed of rapid picture naming, speed of semantic verification, and simple reaction time on a "go-no-go" task. Factor 4 (Declarative Memory) is characterized by total words recalled across five trials and semantic organization of recall on the California Verbal Learning Test. Measures loading on Factor 5 (Motor Speed) include right hand performance time on the Grooved Pegboard and total time on the motor sequencing task. There are 21%, 25%, 23%, 18%, and 13% common variance accounted for by the five factors, respectively.

As presented in Table 4, at least three measures obtained significant loadings on Factors 1 through 3, with two measures each loading on Factors 4 and 5. Measures obtained relatively high loadings on only one factor and low loadings on the other four, suggesting that measures loading on a specific factor share in the construct associated with it but not the other four. The severely injured patients were impaired on all of the measures relative to the mild-to-moderate injury group.

An intercorrelation matrix for the five-factor scores disclosed that all but two correlation coefficients were .50 or higher, the exceptions being the correlation between Factor 1 (discourse) and Factor 5 (motor speed; −0.27) and the correlation between Factor 4 (declarative memory) and Factor 5 (−0.38).

TABLE 4
Factor Loadings of 20 Measures Included in an Exploratory
Factor Analysis Based on Data Obtained From 104 Typically Developing
Children and Assessment of 286 Head Injured Children at Least 36
Months Postinjury

Variable	Discourse (Factor 1)	Problem Solving (Factor 2)	Processing Speed (Factor 3)	Declarative Memory (Factor 4)	Motor Speed (Factor 5)
Core	**89**	1	4	−1	−3
Gist	**86**	1	8	−3	−1
Episode	**82**	5	2	−4	5
PPVT–R	**58**	0	−12	16	−3
WCST	12	**55**	−12	13	4
Twenty questions	18	**43**	13	7	4
Verbal fluency	6	**50**	16	10	−7
Design fluency	1	**44**	27	1	5
Metamemory	10	**37**	1	25	−1
Porteus	1	**59**	17	−6	8
TOL	−1	**52**	−22	4	−13
Divided attention	−2	**48**	22	−5	−19
Coding	−3	31	**60**	0	5
Rapid naming	−7	−14	**−57**	−3	8
Verification speed	−2	15	**−60**	−27	−3
Reaction time	1	13	**−61**	4	0
CVLT total	4	11	2	**72**	−8
CVLT cluster	2	5	5	**76**	6
Grooved pebgoard	0	−1	9	1	**78**
Motor sequencing	−1	−4	−24	−2	**68**

Note. Printed values are multiplied by 100 and rounded to the nearest integer. Values ³ 0.35 are in bold. * PPVT–R = Peabody Picture Vocabulary Test–Revised; WCST = Wisconsin Card Sorting Test; TOL = Tower of London; CVLT = California Verbal Learning Test.

Confirmatory and Exploratory Factor Analyses of the 3-Month Data (Prospective Sample)

Confirmatory factor analysis.   Having produced a five-factor solution to an exploratory factor analysis based on the data of typically developing children and children with TBI who were at least 3 years postinjury, a confirmatory factor analysis was used to test the fit of the five-factor model to data obtained from 265 children in the prospective cohort who were tested 3 months postinjury. In addition to fitness of the model, its convergent and discriminant validity was also examined. The five-factor model provided a reasonably good fit to the 3-month data. The chi-square/*df* ratio (221.57/160 = 1.38) was less than 2, indicating that the model may be acceptable. Values for the Bentler's Comparative Fit Index or CFI (Bentler, 1989) and the Nonnormed Fit Index (NNFI) of Bentler and Bonett (Bentler & Bonett, 1980) were 0.96 and 0.95, respectively, indicating that the five-factor model provided an acceptable fit. Standardized loadings of the 20 measures on the five factors were moderately large, ranging from 0.51 to 0.98, with only five being under 0.60. The distribution of the normalized residuals was centered on zero, but contained some large residuals, suggesting that some of the measures were influenced by more than one factor.

Reliability of the outcome measures was assessed by squaring the standardized factor loadings. Reliabilities ranged from 0.26 to 0.96, with the majority being between 0.5 and 0.9. The composite reliability index for each factor was calculated: Factor 1 (Discourse) = 0.80; Factor 2 (Problem Solving) = 0.75; Factor 3 (Processing Speed) = 0.60; Factor 4 (Declarative Memory) = 0.85; Factor 5 (Motor Speed) = 0.35. Factor 3 (Processing Speed) just met the usual minimally acceptable level of reliability, 0.60 to 0.70; Factor 5 (Motor Speed) was below, indicating that these factors were not sufficiently reliable.

Correlations among the five factors were determined to assess their discriminant validity. The correlations were high, ranging from 0.65 to 0.97, with the highest occurring between Factors 3 (Processing Speed) and 5 (Motor Speed), and Factors 2 (Problem Solving) and 3 (Processing Speed). A confidence interval test of covariance among factors demonstrated a high correlation between Factors 3 (Processing Speed) and 5 (Motor Speed), reflecting a lack of discriminant validity between these factors and suggesting that a number of the measures assessing processing speed and motor speed are associated with the same underlying construct.

Exploratory factor analysis.   Using a method similar to the procedure in the initial exploratory analysis, we analyzed the 3-month data used in the aforementioned confirmatory factor analysis. The final model, which provided the best fit for the 3-month data, was a four-factor model presented in Table 5. To follow the interpretability criteria and the simple structure rule, four measures were dropped from this four-factor model, including Wisconsin Card Sort percent of conceptual

TABLE 5
Factor Loadings of 16 Measures Included in an Exploratory Factor
Analysis Based on Data Obtained From 265 Head Injured Children 3
Months Postinjury

Variable	Discourse (Factor 1)	Problem Solving (Factor 2)	Processing Speed (Factor 3)	Declarative Memory (Factor 4)
Core	**90**	13	8	1
Gist	**82**	1	–4	–1
Episode	**71**	–17	–26	–4
PPVT–R	**52**	7	15	14
Twenty questions	19	**45**	4	9
Verbal fluency	10	**51**	–9	22
Design fluency	6	**64**	–9	4
Porteus	–10	**63**	–8	7
Divided attention	–5	**86**	2	–4
Coding	14	**56**	–20	–4
Rapid naming	–10	–23	**54**	–9
Reaction time	1	8	**71**	–4
Grooved pebgoard	–1	–27	**56**	14
Motor sequencing	6	–10	**50**	–10
CVLT total	4	13	–17	**67**
CVLT cluster	5	7	5	**76**

Note.   Values ≥ 0.35 are in bold. PPVT–R = Peabody Picture Vocabulary Test–Revised; CVLT = California Verbal Learning Test.

responses, a metamemory task, and semantic verification speed, which did not load significantly on any factor, and Tower of London percent solved in three trials, which loaded on Factor 4 (Declarative Memory) instead of Factor 2 (Problem Solving). This four-factor model accounts for the following percentage of the common variance: Factor 1 (Discourse) = 78%; Factor 2 (Problem Solving) = 13%; Factor 3 (Processing–Motor Speed) = 7%; and Factor 4 (Declarative Memory) = 5%. The measures included in this model have high factor loadings on only one factor, indicating that they share in the construct associated only with that factor. As in the five-factor model, discourse measures associated with essential meaning and a measure of receptive vocabulary are associated with Factor 1 (Discourse). Three types of measures are associated with Factor 2 (Problem Solving): (a) measures involving planning and problem solving such as the ability to generate efficient questions and complete complex mazes; (b) measures associated with productivity and self-regulation such as rapid word production and drawing of abstract designs containing four lines according to defined rules; and (c) measures requiring allocation of resources and processing speed such as finger tapping with a distraction and rapid graphomotor transcription of forms on WISC–R Coding.

Measures loading on Factor 3 (Processing–Motor Speed) include Rapid Naming, Reaction Time, Grooved Pegboard, and Motor Sequencing and are associated with productivity and motor speed. Similar to the five-factor model, Factor 4 (Declarative Memory) includes measures involving learning and recall of semantically related word lists. Analysis of TBI severity disclosed that severely injured children were impaired on all measures, with the exception of nonsignificant group differences on the Peabody Picture Vocabulary Test–Revised standard score, the Twenty Questions Test (percent of constraint questions), and movement sequence (total time to complete sequences).

Relation of Severity of Injury to Cognitive Functioning

To assess the sensitivity of the factor scores to variables associated with outcome of TBI in children, analyses of covariance were performed on the exploratory factor-based scores obtained at least 36 months postinjury (Table 6) and at 3 months after injury (Table 7). Severity of injury (mild–moderate vs. severe) was the between-subjects factor and age at testing was used as a covariate. As summarized in Tables 6 and 7, severity of injury and age at testing were significant for the five factors obtained for the 36-month data as well as the four factors obtained for the 3-month data. The interaction of injury severity with age was not significant for any factor, although a trend was observed with the 36-month data for Factor 5 (Motor Speed). A similar analysis substituting age at injury for age at testing also disclosed no interaction of age with TBI severity.

Relation of Cognitive Factors to Adaptive Functioning

To assess the relation between the cognitive factor scores and adaptive functioning, Spearman rank order correlation coefficients were computed based on the data collected at least 36 months postinjury and the 3-month data and mean percentile scores on the Vineland Adaptive Behavior Scales–Revised obtained on the same occasion. This measure assesses the child's functioning in the everyday environment and is based on parent or caretaker report (Sparrow, Balla, & Cicchetti, 1984).

For the data obtained at least 36 months postinjury, Spearman rank order correlation coefficients were significant for the Adaptive Behavior Composite, Communication, Socialization, Daily Living Domain scores, and all five factors. Moderate correlations were obtained for Factor 1 (Discourse) and the Adaptive Behavior Composite ($r = 0.39$, $p < .0001$), Communication ($r = 0.39$, $p < .0001$), Socialization ($r = 0.29$, $p < .0008$), and the Daily Living ($r = 0.26$, $p < .0026$). Moderate correlations were also obtained for Factor 2 (Problem Solving) and the Adaptive Behavior Composite ($r = 0.40$, $p < .0001$), Communication ($r = 0.46$, $p < .0001$), Socialization ($r = 0.26$, $p < .003$), and Daily Living ($r =$

TABLE 6
Analyses of Covariance Performed on the Factor-Based Scores Obtained for the Assessments Completed at Least 36 Months Postinjury (Prospective Cohort)

Factor	Severity (S)		Age at Test (A)		S * A		Mild–Moderate	Severe
	F	p	F	p	F	p		
1	$F(1, 196) = 16.80$	.0001	$F(1, 196) = 40.20$	.0001	$F(1, 196) = 0.20$	.65	0.56 (0.31)	−1.32 (0.32)
2	$F(1, 208) = 20.46$	.0001	$F(1, 208) = 166.93$	.0001	$F(1, 208) = 0.96$	.33	1.00 (0.22)	−0.58 (0.24)
3	$F(1, 191) = 12.81$	.0004	$F(1, 191) = 135.72$	.0001	$F(1, 191) = 2.25$	.14	0.49 (0.20)	−0.66 (0.22)
4	$F(1, 271) = 31.95$	.0001	$F(1, 271) = 66.91$	.0001	$F(1, 271) = 0.08$	.78	0.57 (0.14)	−0.64 (0.15)
5	$F(1, 234) = 9.34$	.003	$F(1, 234) = 20.20$	.0001	$F(1, 234) = 3.64$	.06	−0.36 (0.15)	0.41 (0.17)

Note. Values in parentheses are standard deviations.

TABLE 7

Analyses of Covariance Performed on the Factor-Based Scores Obtained for the Assessments Completed at 3 Months Postinjury

Factor	Severity (S)		Age at Test (A)		S * A		Mild–Moderate	Severe
	F	p	F	p	F	p		
1	$F(1, 179) = 10.55$	.001	$F(1, 179) = 362.37$	.0001	$F(1, 179) = 0.51$	0.47	0.65 (0.22)	−0.62 (0.32)
2	$F(1, 135) = 5.84$	.02	$F(1, 135) = 14.34$	.0001			−0.49 (0.41)	−1.09 (0.57)
3	$F(1, 182) = 12.34$	.0006	$F(1, 182) = 213.03$	.0001	$F(1, 182) = 1.16$	0.28	0.59 (0.32)	−0.78 (0.46)
4	$F(1, 253) = 8.89$	.0001	$F(1, 253) = 106.60$	.0001	$F(1, 253) = 0.31$	0.58	−0.62 (0.18)	0.50 (0.27)

Note. Values in parentheses are standard deviations.

0.23, $p < .0069$). Factor 3 (Processing Speed) correlations ranged from moderate to moderately low, that is, Adaptive Behavior Composite ($r = 0.36$, $p < .0001$), Communication ($r = 0.44$, $p < .0001$), Socialization ($r = 0.23$, $p < .01$), and Daily Living ($r = 0.20$, $p < .02$). Factor 4 (Declarative Memory) had moderate correlations, that is, Adaptive Behavior ($r = 0.48$, $p < 0001$), Communication ($r = 0.39$, $p < .0001$), Socialization ($r = 0.37$, $p < .0001$), and Daily Living ($r = 0.41$, $p < .0001$). Factor 5 (Motor Speed) obtained moderately low correlations with Communication ($r = 0.34$, $p < .0001$ and $r = 0.33$, $p < .0001$).

Separate computation of the Spearman correlations for the patients who sustained mild to moderate head injury disclosed generally nonsignificant results with the exception of the Communication Domain for which correlations with Factors 1–3 were significant, but low. In contrast, correlations for the severely injured children were consistently significant, ranging from 0.27 to 0.54. For the 3-month data, Spearman correlation coefficients were generally nonsignificant with the exception of Factor 4 (Declarative Memory) with Adaptive Behavior Composite ($r = .44$, $p < .0001$), Communication ($r = 0.41$, $p < .0001$), Socialization ($r = 0.33$, $p < .002$), and Daily Living ($r = 0.29$, $p < .001$). Corresponding correlations for the mild to moderately injured children were nonsignificant with the exception of the correlations between Factor 4 (Declarative Memory) and the Adaptive Behavior ($r = 0.32$, $p < .009$), and Communication ($r = 0.37$, $p < .002$). For the children with severe head injury, significant correlations of the 3-month data were also confined to Factor 4 (Declarative Memory) with Adaptive Behavior ($r = 0.50$, $p < .02$) and Communication ($r = 0.42$, $p < .04$).

DISCUSSION

Our findings indicate that EF tests have a meaningful structure and that the factors so derived are related to both the severity of pediatric TBI and to adaptive functioning at 3 years postinjury. Although limitations of this study are noted later, we suggest that the factor scores may be useful for data-reduction purposes and in clinical trials.

With a lack of consensus on delineating EFs in children, factor analysis offers an empirical approach to characterizing the key dimensions of these abilities. In addition to children sustaining TBI, this research is relevant to other pediatric populations with EF deficits, including children with autism, attention-deficit–hyperactivity disorder (Barkley, 1997), early treated phenylketonuria (Diamond, Prevor, Callender, & Druin, 1997), and Fragile X Syndrome (Mazzocco, Pennington, & Hagerman, 1993). Our series of EF measures differs from most previous studies by including narrative discourse, in which we analyzed the child's capacity to extract the essential or "gist" information from a fable. Although we had conceptualized the ability to summarize and extract key information as a supraordinate skill involving EFs, the discourse processing and PPVT–R standard score loaded on a factor that could be parsimoniously interpreted as verbal ability. However, the highest loadings of Factor 1 were on the discourse measures, which putatively involved working memory for the salient aspects of the stories and inhibition of unimportant details. Although the finding of a verbal factor is consistent with Goldman-Rakic's proposal (Goldman-Rakic, 1998) that representation of working memory in dorsolateral prefrontal cortex is organized primarily by information content, this view would not explain the Factor 2 loadings, which include measures that are heterogeneous in content such as shapes and colors (e.g., Wisconsin Card Sorting Test) and words generated on the phonemic fluency test.

Cognitive operations, including flexibility in problem solving, planning, and allocation of attentional resources appear to better define Factor 2 than the content being manipulated. Although these operations differ somewhat in processing demands, they all involve cognitive control, which is ostensibly mediated by prefrontally guided, distributed networks (Miller & Cohen, 2001) that are vulnerable to diffuse axonal injury and focal lesions of prefrontal cortex (Adams et al., 1980). Consistent with our measure of metamemory probing use of strategy, cognitive flexibility, and organizational skills rather than testing long-term recall or recognition, it loaded primarily on Factor 2 instead of the declarative memory factor. Our finding that declarative memory, as measured by the CVLT, loaded on a separate factor is consistent with focal brain lesion (Petrides, 2000) and functional brain imaging (Braver et al., 2001) studies indicating that working memory and declarative memory are interactive abilities with at least partially distinct cortical representations.

Consistent with the partition of problem solving and declarative memory by the factor analysis, focal frontal lesions in children can disproportionately impair executive functions including emotional regulation with relative preservation of performance on declarative memory tests (Anderson, Damasio, Tranel, & Damasio, 2000). Although processing speed might not be considered an EF, we included measures of this domain because of its interaction with abilities such as problem solving and working memory, which are negatively impacted by slower processing speed (Roberts & Pennington, 1996). For purposes of divergent validity, two measures of motor speed were also included in this study.

Cognitive theorists have posited a relation between processing speed and demands on working memory (Barkley, 1997). However, the distinction between Factors 2 and 3 may be based on monitoring–manipulation of information and complexity of problem solving (Wisconsin Card Sort, Porteus Mazes, Tower of London) as opposed to rapid performance of well-established skills such as retrieval from semantic memory (Verification Speed) and lexical access (Rapid Naming). Our finding that declarative memory (as measured by the CVLT) loaded on a separate factor relative to problem solving is consistent with focal brain lesion (Petrides, 2000) studies indicating that working memory and declarative memory are interactive abilities that have at least partially distinct cortical representations. Consistent with the partition of problem solving and declarative memory by the factor analysis, focal frontal lesions in children can disproportionately impair executive cognitive functions and emotional regulation with relative preservation of declarative memory (Anderson et al., 2000). Similarly, Factor 4 was composed of a test of declarative memory that does not primarily involve shifting of mental set, manipulation of information, and problem solving. Using long-term outcome data collected at 36 months or longer postinjury, we found that measures of motor speed (Factor 5) were differentiated from cognitive processing speed (Factor 4). In contrast, cognitive processing and motor speed measures both loaded on a single factor in an exploratory factor analysis of the 3-month outcome data, possibly reflecting marked, generalized slowing of performance, which is characteristic of children during the early phase of recovery from severe TBI.

The current factor solutions differ from our preliminary findings (Levin, Fletcher, Kufera, et al., 1996), which were based on a smaller sample of patients and a narrower set of variables. Despite the differences, in both studies the WCST and fluency measures loaded on the same factor, and a separate factor was defined by the CVLT cluster measure. With a larger number of variables per factor and a larger sample size, the current factor structure is more reliable than the solution obtained in the preliminary study. The effect of TBI severity on factor scores was also more consistent in this study as compared with the previous investigation.

Based on experimental studies of prefrontal cortical ablation effects on delayed alternation performance in monkeys, Goldman (1974) posited that dorsolateral and orbitofrontal lesion effects differed depending on the animal's age at injury. Based on Goldman's seminal work, it is plausible that the immediate effects of injury to specific prefrontal subregions when they are functionally immature might not be initially apparent, with later effects being observed when these anatomic regions typically reach functional maturity. The finding that synaptic pruning in human prefrontal cortex occurs during late adolescence relative to earlier maturation of other cortical regions (Huttenlocher & Dabholkar, 1997) is compatible with this view of injury effects. These findings lead to the prediction in this study of an interaction between age at injury and TBI severity. However, we did not find an interaction between age at testing or at time of injury and TBI severity.

These findings are applicable to clinical trials of interventions for pediatric TBI. The loading of measures in this study provides a better understanding of the underlying constructs being assessed, thus providing a basis for selection of specific outcome measures to assess EFs of interest. Utilization of factor scores would allow for the reduction of the number of outcome measures and facilitate data reduction. Our finding that factor scores obtained at least 36 months postinjury were related to a well-established measure of adaptive functioning (Vineland Adaptive Behavior Scales–Revised, Sparrow et al., 1984) provides support for the validity of this approach. Although the relation between factor scores at 3 months postinjury and adaptive functioning was relatively weak, this postinjury interval might have been insufficient to assess the impact of EF deficits on various domains of psychosocial adjustment. Further investigation could determine the relation of the factor scores to other outcome and behavioral measures such as the Glasgow Outcome Scale (Jennett & Bond, 1975), the Behavioral Assessment System for Children (Reynolds & Kamphaus, 1998; Vaughn, Riccio, Hynd, & Hall, 1997), and the Behavioral Rating Inventory of Executive Function (Gioia, Isquith, Guy, & Kenworthy, 2000).

ACKNOWLEDGMENTS

Research presented in this article was supported by Grant NS–21889 from the National Institute of Neurological Disorders and Stroke.
We are indebted to Angela D. Williams for editorial assistance.

REFERENCES

Adams, J. H., Graham, D. I., Scott, G., Parker, L. S., & Doyle, D. (1980). Brain damage in fatal non-missile head injury. *Journal of Clinical Pathology, 33,* 1132–1145.

Anderson, S. W., Damasio, H., Tranel, D., & Damasio, A. R. (2000). Long-term sequelae of prefrontal cortex damage acquired in early childhood. *Developmental Neuropsychology, 18,* 281–296.

Anderson, V., Levin, H. S., & Jacobs, R. (2002). Executive functions following frontal lobe injury: A developmental perspective. In D. T. Stuss & R. T. Knight (Eds.), *Principles of frontal lobe function* (pp. 504–527). New York: Oxford University Press.

Baddeley, A., & Wilson, B. (1988). Frontal amnesia and the dysexecutive syndrome. *Brain Cognition, 7,* 212–230.

Barkley, R. A. (1997). Behavioral inhibition, sustained attention, and executive functions: Constructing a unifying theory of ADHD. *PsychologicalBulletin, 121,* 65–94.

Bentler, P. M. (1989). EQS Structural Equations Program [Computer software]. Los Angeles: BMOP Statistical Software.

Bentler, P. M., & Bonett, D. G. (1980). Significance tests and goodness of fit in the analysis of covariance structures. *Psychological Bulletin, 88,* 588–606.

Benton, A. L. (1968). Differential behavioral effects in frontal lobe disease. *Neuropsychologia, 6,* 53–60.

Borkowski, J. G., & Burke, J. E. (1996). Theories, models, and measurements of executive functioning: An information processing perspective. In G. R. Lyon & N. A. Krasnegor (Eds.), *Attention, Memory, and Executive Function* (pp. 235–262). Baltimore: Brookes.

Braver, T. S., Barch, D. M., Kelley, W. M., Buckner, R. L., Cohen, N. J., Miezin, F. M., et al. (2001). Direct comparison of prefrontal cortex regions engaged by working and long-term memory tasks. *Neuroimage., 14,* 48–59.

Cabeza, R., & Nyberg, L. (2000). Imaging cognition II: An empirical review of 275 PET and fMRI studies. *Journal of Cognitive Neuroscience, 21,* 1–47.

Casey, B. J., Castellanos, F. X., Giedd, J. N., Marsh, W. L., Hamburger, S. D., Schubert, A. B., et al. (1997). Implication of right frontostriatal circuitry in response inhibition and attention-deficit/hyperactivity disorder. *Journal of the American Academy of Child and Adolescent Psychiatry, 36,* 374–383.

Chapman, S. B., Culhane, K. A., Levin, H. S., Harward, H., Mendelsohn, D., Ewing-Cobbs, L., et al. (1992). Narrative discourse after closed head injury in children and adolescents. *Brain & Language, 43,* 42–65.

Delis, D. C., Kramer, J. H., Kaplan, E., & Ober, B. A. (1986). *The California Verbal Learning Test–research edition.* New York: Psychological Corporation.

Denckla, M. B. (1996). A theory and model of executive function: A neuropsychological perspective. In G. R. Lyon & N. A. Krasnegor (Eds.), *Attention, memory, and executive function* (pp. 263–279). Baltimore: Brookes.

Denckla, M. B., & Rudel, R. (1974). Rapid automatized naming of pictured objects, colors, letters, and numbers by normal children. *Cortex, 10,* 184–202.

Denney, D. R., & Denney, N. W. (1973). The use of classification for problem-solving: A comparison of middle and old age. *Developmental Psychology, 9,* 275–278.

Dennis, M., Barnes, M. A., Wilkinson, M., & Humphreys, R. P. (1998). How children with head injury represent real and deceptive emotion in short narratives. *Brain & Language, 61,* 450–483.

Dennis, M., & Lovett, M. W. (1990). Discourse ability in children after brain damage. In Y.Joanette & H. H. Brownell (Eds.), *Discourse ability and brain damage: Theoretical and empirical perspectives* (pp. 199–223). New York: Springer-Verlag.

Diamond, A. (1991). Guidelines for the study of brain-behavior relationships during development. In H. S. Levin, H. M. Eisenberg, & A. L. Benton (Eds.), *Frontal lobe function and dysfunction* (pp. 339–378). New York: Oxford University Press.

Diamond, A., Prevor, M. B., Callender, G., & Druin, D. P. (1997). Prefrontal cortex cognitive deficits in children treated early and continuously for PKU. *Monographs of the Society for Research in Child Development, 62,* i-208.

Drewe, E. A. (1975). Go-no go learning after frontal lobe lesions in humans. *Cortex, 11,* 8–16.

Duncan, J. (1986). Disorganization of behaviour after frontal lobe damage. *Cognitive Neuropsychology, 3,* 271–290.

Dunn, L. M., & Dunn, L. M. (1981). *Peabody Picture Vocabulary Test–Revised.* Circle Pines, MN: American Guidance Service.

Eslinger, P. J., Grattan, L. M., Damasio, H., & Damasio, A. R. (1992). Developmental consequences of childhood frontal lobe damage. *Archives of Neurology, 49,* 764–769.

Giedd, J. N., Snell, J. W., Lange, N., Rajapakse, J. C., Casey, B. J., Kozuch, P. L., et al. (1996). Quantitative magnetic resonance imaging of human brain development: Ages 4–18. *Cerebral Cortex, 6,* 551–560.

Gioia, G. A., Isquith, P. K., Guy, S. C., & Kenworthy, L. (2000). *Behavior rating inventory of executive function.* Odessa, FL: Psychological Assessment Resources.

Goldman, P. S. (1974). An alternative to developmental plasticity: Heterology of CNS structures in infants and adults. In D. G. Instein, J. Rosen, & N. Butters (Eds.), *CNS plasticity and recovery of function* (pp. 149–174). New York: Academic.

Goldman-Rakic, P. S. (1998). The prefrontal landscape: Implications of functional architecture for understanding human mentation and the central executive. In A. C. Roberts, T. W. Robbins, & L. Weiskrantz (Eds.), *The prefrontal cortex* (pp. 87–102). Oxford, UK: Oxford University Press.

Grafman, J., & Litvan, I. (1999). Importance of deficits in executive functions. *Lancet, 354,* 1921–1923.

Graham, S., & Harris, K. R. (1996). Addressing problems in attention, memory, and executive functioning: An example from self-regulated strategy development. In G. R. Lyon & N. A. Krasnegor (Eds.), *Attention, memory, and executive function* (pp. 349–366). Baltimore: Brookes.

Grant, D. A., & Berg, E. A. (1948). A behavioral analysis of degree of reinforcement and ease of shifting to new responses in a Weigl-type card-sorting problem. *Journal of Experimental Psychology, 38,* 404–411.

Heaton, R. K., Chelune, G. J., Talley, J. L., Kay, G. G., & Curtis, G. (1993). *Wisconsin Card Sorting Test (WCST) manual revised and expanded.* Odessa, FL: Psychological Assessment Resources.

Hiscock, M., Kinsbourne, M., Samuels, M., & Krause, A. E. (1987). Dual task performance in children: Generalized and lateralized effects of memory encoding upon the rate and variability of concurrent finger tapping. *Brain & Cognition, 6,* 24–40.

Huttenlocher, P. R., & Dabholkar, A. S. (1997). Regional differences in synaptogenesis in human cerebral cortex. *Journal of Comparative Neurology, 387,* 167–178.

Jennett, B., & Bond, M. (1975). Assessment of outcome after severe brain damage. A practical scale. *Lancet, 1,* 480–487.

Jones-Gotman, M., & Milner, B. (1977). Design fluency: The invention of nonsense drawings after focal cortical lesions. *Neuropsychologia, 15,* 653–674.

Levin, H. S., Culhane, K. A., Fletcher, J. M., Mendelsohn, D. B., Lilly, M. A., Harward, H., et al. (1994). Dissociation between delayed alternation and memory after pediatric head injury: Relationship to MRI findings. *Journal of Child Neurology, 9,* 81–89.

Levin, H. S., Culhane, K. A., Mendelsohn, D., Lilly, M. A., Bruce, D., Fletcher, J. H. M., et al. (1993). Cognition in relation to magnetic resonance imaging in head injured children and adolescents. *Archives of Neurology, 50,* 897–905.

Levin, H. S., Eisenberg, H. M., Wigg, N. R., & Kobayashi, K. (1982). Memory and intellectual ability after head injury in children and adolescents. *Neurosurgery, 11,* 668–673.

Levin, H. S., Fletcher, J. M., Kufera, J. A., Harward, H., Lilly, M. A., Mendelsohn, D., et al. (1996). Dimensions of cognition measured by the Tower of London and other cognitive tasks in head-injured children and adolescents. *Developmental Neuropsychology, 12,* 17–34.

Levin, H. S., Fletcher, J. M., Kusnerik, L., Kufera, J., Lilly, M. A., Duffy, F. F., et al. (1996). Semantic memory following pediatric head injury: Relationship to age, severity of injury, and MRI. *Cortex, 32,* 461–478.

Levin, H. S., Mendelsohn, D., Lilly, M. A., Fletcher, J. M., Culhane, K. A., Chapman, S. B., et al. (1994). Tower of London performance in relation to magnetic resonance imaging following closed head injury in children. *Neuropsychology, 8,* 171–179.

Levin, H. S., Mendelsohn, D., Lilly, M. A., Yeakley, J., Song, J., Scheibel, R. S., et al. (1997). Magnetic resonance imaging in relation to functional outcome of pediatric closed head injury: A test of the Ommaya-Gennarelli model. *Neurosurgery, 40,* 432–440.

Levin, H. S., Song, J., Ewing-Cobbs, L., & Roberson, G. (2001). Porteus Maze performance following traumatic brain injury in children. *Neuropsychology, 15,* 557–567.

Luciana, M., & Nelson, C. A. (1998). The functional emergence of prefrontally-guided working memory systems in four- to eight-year-old children. *Neuropsychologia, 36,* 273–293.

Luria, A. R. (1966). *Higher cortical functions in man.* New York: Basic Books.

Marlowe, W. (1992). The impact of right prefrontal lesion on the developing brain. *Brain and Cognition, 20,* 205–213.

Matthews, C. G., & Kløve, H. (1964). *Instruction manual for the Adult Neuropsychology Test Battery.* Madison, WI: University of Wisconsin Medical School.

Mazzocco, M. M., Pennington, B. F., & Hagerman, R. J. (1993). The neurocognitive phenotype of female carriers of fragile X: additional evidence for specificity. *Journal of Developmental and Behavioral Pediatrics, 14,* 328–335.

Miller, E. K. (2000). The prefrontal cortex: No simple matter. *Neuroimage, 11,* 447–450.

Miller, E. K., & Cohen, J. D. (2001). An integrative theory of prefrontal cortex function. *Annual Review of Neuroscience, 24,* 167–202.

Pennington, B. F., Bennetto, L., McAleer, O., & Roberts, R. J., Jr. (1996). Executive functions and working memory: Theoretical and measurement issues. In G. R. Lyon & N. A. Krasnegor (Eds.), *Attention, memory, and executive function* (pp. 327–348). Baltimore: Brookes.

Petrides, M. (2000). The role of the mid-dorsolateral prefrontal cortex in working memory. *Experimental Brain Research, 133,* 44–54.

DEVELOPMENTAL NEUROPSYCHOLOGY, 25(1&2), 85–106

Childhood Head Injury and Metacognitive Processes in Language and Memory

Gerri Hanten
Cognitive Neuroscience Laboratory
Department of Physical Medicine and Rehabilitation
Baylor College of Medicine
Houston, TX

Maureen Dennis
Department of Psychology
Hospital for Sick Children
Toronto, Ontario, Canada

Lifang Zhang
Cognitive Neuroscience Laboratory
Department of Physical Medicine and Rehabilitation
Baylor College of Medicine
Houston, TX

Marcia Barnes
Department of Psychology
Hospital for Sick Children
Toronto, Ontario, Canada

Garland Roberson
Cognitive Neuroscience Laboratory
Department of Physical Medicine and Rehabilitation
Baylor College of Medicine
Houston, TX

Requests for reprints should be sent to Gerri Hanten, Cognitive Neuroscience Laboratory, Baylor College of Medicine, 6560 Fannin Street, Ste. 1144, Box 67, Houston, TX 77030. E-mail: ghanten@bcm.tmc.edu

Jennifer Archibald
Department of Psychology
Hospital for Sick Children
Toronto, Ontario, Canada

James Song
Department of Biometry
Bayer Pharmaceuticals
New Haven, CT

Harvey S. Levin
Cognitivie Neuroscience Laboratory
Departments of Physical Medicine and Rehabilitation,
Neurosurgery, and Psychiatry and Behavioral Sciences
Baylor College of Medicine
Houston, TX

We studied the metacognitive functioning of children with severe and mild traumatic brain injury (TBI) and typically developing children. To test metacognition for memory, children were tested on a modified Judgment of Learning task. We found that children with severe TBI were impaired in their ability to predict recall of specific items prior to study–recall trials, but were unimpaired in predicting recall on a delayed test when the judgment was made after study–recall trials. Metacognitive knowledge impairment for memorial abilities was also demonstrated in children with severe TBI by poor estimation of memory span and exaggerated overconfidence in performance. To test metacognition within the language domain, we gave children a sentence anomaly detection and repair task in which spoken sentences were monitored for semantic anomalies. Children with severe TBI were impaired on the detection of semantic anomalies, especially under conditions of high memory load. However, metalinguistic knowledge in the form of adequate repairs of anomalous sentences, was preserved. Results are discussed in terms of effects of age at test and injury severity.

The ability to observe, evaluate, and exert control over our own mental processes is considered a uniquely human characteristic. The term *metacognition*, literally cognition about one's own cognition, is applied to this self-reflective aspect of our cognitive processes.

In recent years theorists have come to substantial agreement that metacognition is multicomponent, comprising (at minimum) metacognitive monitoring, metacognitive control, and metacognitive knowledge (Mazzoni & Nelson, 1998; Metcalfe & Shimamura, 1994; Nelson, 1992). Metacognitive monitoring includes conscious awareness and evaluation of ongoing cognitive processes such as the determination of whether or not one understands a particular sentence, or the evaluation of whether a mnemonic strategy is proving effective, or the assessment of one's progress on a particular task. Metacognitive control includes the self-regulatory and management aspects of cognition (Mazzoni & Nelson, 1998), and, according to some theorists, may include those aspects of cognitive control that are not necessarily subject to conscious awareness, but are auto-regulated. Examples of cognitive control include the selective inhibition of irrelevant information during task performance, the application of particular strategies in problem solving, or appropriate resource allocation in the accomplishment of a task (Brown, 1978; Brown & DeLoache, 1978). Metacognitive knowledge refers to the information accumulated over time about one's own abilities, state of knowledge, and resources. It would seem that such abilities would be critical to development of the skills and knowledge necessary for satisfactory scholastic achievement and to function independently.

METACOGNITION IN TYPICALLY DEVELOPING CHILDREN

Metacognition has a protracted developmental course. Research studies show that overall competence increases with age, and, further, that the different components of metacognition have somewhat different developmental timeframes (Schneider, 1998).

Metacognitive abilities in children appear to start to develop at an early age, though there is variation in the age at which different abilities appear. Early studies within the memory domain, for example, found that young children do recognize that an instruction to remember requires a special effort, but until around 7 years of age, they do not come up with especially effective strategies (Appel et al., 1972; Flavell, Beach, & Chinsky, 1966; Garrity, 1975). Preschoolers are aware of the increased difficulty of remembering items over longer time periods, but not until around age 8 do they implement longer study times in response to longer retention intervals (Rogoff, Newcombe, & Kagan, 1974), leading to a decrease in errors. Similarly, though young children can distinguish between difficult and easy items to remember, unlike older children, they do not allocate more study time to these items (Dufresne & Kobasigawa, 1989).

The development of successful metacognition appears to be associated with increased competence in other cognitive domains. The self-regulatory or metacognitive control activities that are most closely associated with the central executive in information processing models of cognition, particularly working memory, seem to begin to develop early in childhood (Brown, 1978; Brown & DeLoache, 1978). By about the age of 6 or 7, children start to use rehearsal as a memorization strategy (Keeney, Cannizzo, & Flavell, 1967; Kennedy & Miller, 1976) and by around the age of 9 they have acquired the concept that categorization can help memorization (Moynahan, 1973; Worden & Sladewski-Awig, 1982). Regarding self-assessment, young grade-school children have been consistently found to overestimate their own memory spans, with the degree of overestimation decreasing with age (Flavell, Friedrichs, & Hoyt, 1970; Wellman, Collins, & Glieberman, 1981). However, some conditions within a task also seem to affect metacognitive judgments across age groups. For example, children of all ages are better at making judgments of their own recall abilities based on aggregates of stimulus items rather than on individual items (Schneider, Visé, Lockl, & Nelson, 2000).

In the language domain, comparable differences in the development of metacognitive abilities have been observed. For example, young children are able to monitor and recognize ambiguity in the first part of a two-part instruction, but tend to judge the whole instruction as clear if the second part of the instruction was unambiguous, even when it did not resolve the initial ambiguity. In contrast, older participants recognize the need to integrate both parts of an instruction to determine ambiguity (Flavell, Green, & Flavell, 1985). The degree to which such findings might reflect the interaction of language monitoring abilities and memory capacity is not clear. There is some evidence that the developmental change in the ability to monitor spoken prose may be related to the reduced working memory capacity or slower semantic processing of younger children as compared to older children and adults (Holcomb, Coffey, & Neville, 1992; Liu, Bates, Powell, & Wulfeck, 1997; Tyler & Marlsen-Wilson, 1981).

Metacognition in Children With TBI

Children with traumatic brain injury (TBI) have long been described as having difficulty organizing their own life and learning. Part of this difficulty has been linked to impairments in many areas of executive functioning, including inhibitory and interference control, problem solving, selective attention, planning, and discourse processing (Chapman et al., 1997; Dennis, Wilkinson, Koski, & Humphreys, 1995; Ewing-Cobbs et al., 1998; Levin et al., 1996).

Recent research has linked TBI-related cognitive deficits in children to impairment in metacognitive abilities, at least within the domains of language (Dennis, Barnes, Donnelly, Wilkinson, & Humphreys, 1996; Hanten, Levin, & Song, 1999) and memory (Hanten, Bartha, & Levin, 2000). Dennis et al. (1996) reported that children with TBI exhibited impairment on tests of metacognitive abilities (i.e., sentence anomaly detection and repair), particularly when the injuries occurred prior to age 7 and involved contusional damage to the frontal lobe visible on CT scans. In a study of sentence comprehension in severe TBI children who were at least 6 months postinjury, Hanten, Levin, and Song (1999) replicated and extended the findings of Dennis et al. (1996) by investigating the effect of working memory load on detection of sentence anomalies. Hanten et al. found that increased working memory load affected anomaly detection for the TBI children, but not for the uninjured control children. They also found that even when the TBI children and the control children were equated for performance on the sentence anomaly detection task, the TBI children were significantly poorer at repairing anomalous sentences (i.e., rephrasing the sentence to make sense). Evidence from these studies suggests that measurable impairments in metacognition may result from severe pediatric TBI, effects apparently moderated by the presence of frontal lobe lesions and a younger age at injury. Poor metacognitive functioning is common in children after TBI, and may contribute, with other cognitive factors, to the demonstrated deficits in language comprehension, memory, and learning.

To date, studies on metacognition in children with TBI have demonstrated the existence of impairments in this domain. Research with this special population has lagged behind studies of typical development in fractionating the metacognition domain. A better and more specific characterization of the observed metacognitive deficits in children with TBI is important to furthering our understanding of the long-term consequences of this condition. In this article, we review recent progress in understanding metacognitive deficits and their relation to cognitive development in children who have sustained TBI. We report here findings from studies relating to metacognitive processing using tasks from the domains of working memory and language processing. Within these tasks there are components of metacognitive knowledge, monitoring and control, which we analyze in relation to TBI severity and age at test. Of particular interest is the interface between metacognition and cognitive processes such as working memory.

Participants

Participants were at least 3 years post-TBI and were recruited from cohorts established in previous studies that sampled consecutive admissions to Ben Taub General Hospital and Texas Children's Hospital, Baylor College of Medicine, Houston; Hermann Children's Hospital, the University of Houston Medical School at Houston; Children's Medical Center, the University of Texas Southwestern Medical Center, Dallas; The Hospital for Sick Children, Toronto. Children were between the ages of 5 and 15 at the time of testing. Exclusionary criterion included non-English speakers, illegal immigrants, Abbreviated Injury Scale score of 2 or higher for extracranial injury, previous hospitalization for head injury; preexisting neurologic disorder associated with cerebral dysfunction or cognitive deficit (i.e., cerebral palsy, mental retardation, epilepsy), preexisting severe psychiatric disorder (autism, schizophrenia, pervasive developmental disorder), penetrating gunshot wound to the head, injury caused by child abuse, hypoxia, and hypotension. Severity of injury was measured using the lowest postresuscitation Glasgow Coma Scale (GCS) score of Teasdale and Jennett (1974).

Healthy children from the Houston, Dallas, and Toronto communities were recruited to serve as normal controls based on age and similar socioeconomic background.

METACOGNITION AND WORKING MEMORY

Judgment of Learning Task (Hanten et al., 2000; Hanten et al., 1999; Leonesio & Nelson, 1990).

To address the effect of TBI on metacognitive processing within the memory domain, we used a Judgment of Learning Task (JOL) embedded in a multitrial learning and recall task adapted from Leonesio and Nelson (1990). The task comprises three metacognitive judgments and four learning–recall trials on which the metacognitive judgments are based. In normal adults, the JOL has been shown to be predictive of subsequent performance on memory tests (Leonesio & Nelson, 1990). This task requires metacognitive processing on several levels. The participant must estimate the number of items that she or he will recall, predict, or reflect on the state of one's learning of an individual item and integrate the two types of information.

Method

Participants. On this task we tested 37 children with severe TBI (GCS = 3–8), 40 children with mild TBI (GCS = 13–15), and 32 typically developing control children. Table 1 shows age, gender, and injury characteristics for each group. Preliminary analyses indicated that the three groups had similar distributions of age at test, and the means did not differ significantly ($p = .92$) The mild and severe

TABLE 1
Age and Injury Characteristics of Children in the Control, Mild TBI, and
Severe TBI Groups for the Judgment of Learning Task

Group (n)	Mean Age-at-Test in Years (Range)	Mean Age-at-Injury in Years (Range)	Mean Interval Since Injury in Years (Range)	GCS Mean (SD)	Boys (no.)/ Girls (no.)
Control (32)	12.2 (5.5–16.7)	na	na	na	17/15
Mild TBI (40)	12.3 (6.3–16.4)	6.9 (2.6–12.9)	5.6 (2.01–14.9)	14.7 (.62)	26/14
Severe TBI (37)	12.0 (5.1–16.8)	7.2 (2.8–13.6)	4.9 (2.02–11.1)	7.4 (2.9)	23/14

Note. TBI = traumatic brain injury; GCS = Glasgow Coma Scale.

groups did not differ significantly on age at injury ($p = .47$), nor interval since injury ($p = .15$).

Materials and procedure.   Each child was visually presented a list of 15 low imageability, low-age-of-acquisition words to learn. The child was first given the printed list of words and asked to make a prediction as to which words would be learned, called Ease of Learning judgment (EOL), then was given three study-and-recall trials of the printed word list. Study of the list was limited to 45 sec (3 sec per word), but recall was not time limited. The procedure utilized in the study–recall trials was based on findings in a preliminary study (Hanten et al., 2000) and designed to minimize differences in immediate recall between the children with severe TBI and the control children. Following the third recall trial, the child made a second judgment (JOL), which was the child's appraisal of how well a particular item has been learned—that is, whether or not the he or she would be able to recall the item after a 2-hr delay. Finally, following the final delayed recall trial, the child was asked to assess his or her performance on the test by indicating which of the words he or she thought had been correctly recalled—the Judgment of Knowing (JOK). For each of the judgments, the child could make one of three responses: "easy," "hard," or "not sure" for the EOL; "sure I will remember," "sure I will not remember," or "not sure" for the JOL; and "sure I did remember," "sure I did not remember," or "not sure" for the JOK. For each of the judgments, the child was allowed unlimited time.

Data analyses: Because the variables were counting processes or binary outcomes, the assumption of normal distribution for the ordinary general linear models or repeated measures models were not satisfied. Therefore we modeled the outcome with severity group, using age at test as a covariate, by generalized estimating equation (GEE) model. The SAS procedure GENMOD and logit or log link function was used depending on the form of the outcome variables. The GENMOD procedure fits a GEE model to the data by maximum likelihood estimation of the parameter vectors, the statistic of interest being Likelihood Ratio chi-square.

Results

Recall Performance

The recall performance of the three groups (severe TBI, mild TBI, and control) at each recall period was analyzed using one-tailed t test comparisons assuming unequal variances between groups. One-tailed comparisons were justified by a large body of evidence demonstrating that persons with TBI are likely to show impairments in verbal recall performance. Figure 1 shows the mean number of words recalled in each of the learning trials among the groups. Though there appears to be a trend for the severe TBI group to recall fewer words than the two other groups, there were no significant differences among the groups, thus differential levels of recall among groups as an explanatory factor was ruled out. There was an overall effect of age at test, $\chi^2(1, N = 109) = 9.52$, $p = .002$, such that younger children recalled fewer words than did older children, but no interaction with group.

Learning and forgetting.   The learning over study trials was estimated by subtracting words recalled on Trial 1 from words recalled on Trial 3 for each participant. The amount of learning (Trial 3 recall minus Trial 1 recall) and forgetting from the final study to the 2-hr delayed recall test (Trial 3 recall minus Trial 4 recall) was compared between the groups (Figure 2). Because the outcome variables of interest were integer numbers from 0 to 7, Poisson distributions of outcome variables were considered and a generalized linear model was adopted for these analyses. As can been seen in Figure 2, the mean words learned was less for the severe TBI group ($M = 1.79$) than for the other groups (mild, $M = 2.26$; control, $M = 2.18$), but these difference failed to reach significance. There were no other signifi-

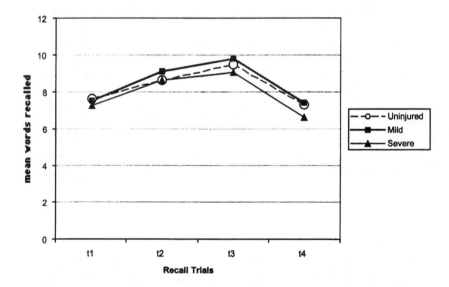

FIGURE 1   Mean words recalled on recall trials by trial and head injury group for the Judgment of Learning Task.

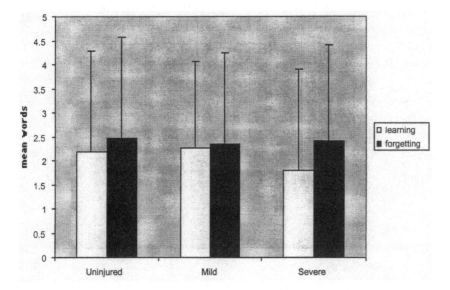

FIGURE 2   Mean number of words and standard deviations (bars) learned from Trial 1 to Trial 3 (learning) and words forgotten from Trial 3 to the delayed Trial 4 (forgetting) by head injury group.

cant differences between groups on learning, and no differences on the measure of forgetting.

Metacognitive Functioning

Metacognitive knowledge: Self-knowledge of memory span.   To estimate the degree of self-knowledge about memory span, we counted the number of words on the EOL judgment that the child had indicated she or he would recall. The number of words from this count was then compared to the number of words that were recalled on Trial 1, without regard to the correspondence between specific items predicted and recalled. In other words, for this measure we compared only the *number* of items that were predicted to be recalled to the number that were recalled, thus gaining an idea of whether or not the child took his or her memory span into account when making the predictions. Generalized linear model with log link function (Poisson regression) was used in this analysis. The outcome (dependent) variable is the number of words over-estimated (i.e., the difference between words predicted and recalled). Independent variables are group, age at test. Analysis revealed that there was a main effect of group, $\chi^2(2, N = 109) = 8.12, p = .01$, and an effect of age at test, $\chi^2(1, N = 109) = 3.67, p = .05$. There was no interaction of group with age at test. Although children in all three groups overestimated the number of words that they would recall

(Figure 3), planned comparisons revealed that the control children overestimated to a lesser degree than did the children with severe TBI, $\chi^2(1, N = 69) = 7.19, p < .01$, or than the children with mild TBI, $\chi^2(1, N = 72) = 5.03, p < .05$; the mild and the severe groups did not differ significantly from each other.

Metacognitive monitoring: Ease of learning, judgment of learning, judgment of knowing. For each participant, the correspondence between a child's prediction for a specific item and whether or not the item was recalled in the delayed recall trial was calculated to give a measure of accuracy of judgment. Items to which the child responded "not sure" were not included in the analyses. For the metacognitive measures we used a generalized linear model with logit link function (logistic regression). Because the outcome variable of interest is the total correct correspondence over the total number of predictions, the logit link function $(\log(p/(1 - p)))$ links the probability of total correspondence to the linear predictor. The accuracy of judgment in terms of proportion correct for each of the three judgments is shown in Figure 4.

EOL. This first judgment was the child's prediction of later performance. This judgment is based on the child's assessment made prior to the learning trials

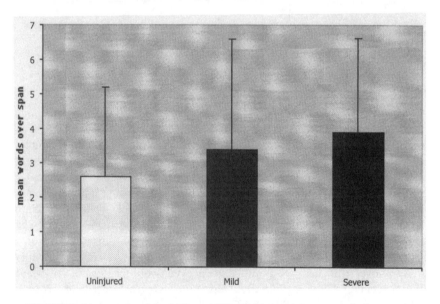

FIGURE 3   Mean number of words (bars = *SD*) by which participants prospectively overestimated their own memory span on Trial 1.

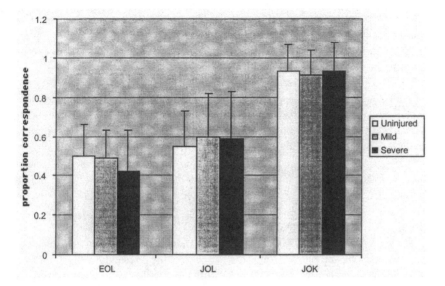

FIGURE 4   Accuracy of judgment in terms of proportion correspondence between judgments and recall on the delayed recall Trial 4 (bars = *SD*).

of his or her ability to recall an item after a 2-hr delay. Overall performance on this measure was fairly low, with mean accuracy across groups only about .47 correct. Children with severe TBI differed significantly from the control children, $\chi^2(1, N = 69) = 4.96, p < .05$, and the children with mild TBI, $\chi^2(1, N = 72) = 4.63, p < .05$. The control and mild groups did not differ significantly from each other on this measure.

JOL.   This second judgment was made by the child after the study and recall trials, and reflects his or her prediction of each item for delayed recall. For this judgment, the child must use the information gained about his or her performance with an item over three study and recall trials and therefore must accurately monitor his or her performance on the recall trials. On this judgment, overall performance for each group was slightly better than for the EOL (*M* = .59), though there were no significant differences among the groups.

JOK.   This third judgment was the child's retrospective evaluation of his or her performance on the delayed recall trial. Accuracy was very high for all three groups on this measure, with performance across groups at better than .90 accuracy. There were no significant differences among the groups. Age at test did not emerge as a significant factor in any of the three judgments.

Confidence.   Given a choice of "easy" to learn or remember or "hard" to learn or remember, we thought that it might be possible that a negative judgment might actually reflect a child's uncertainty of recall, rather than certainty of not learning or remembering. To control for this possibility we allowed a response of "not sure" for each of the ratings. This also allowed us to look at the relative degree of confidence shown by the different groups for each measure using a generalized linear model with logit link function (logistic regression). Because the outcome variable of interest is the total correct correspondence over the total number of predictions, the logit link function ($\log(p/(1 - p))$) links the probability of total correspondence to the linear predictor. When the proportion of "not sure" judgments were calculated for each child for each judgment, we found that only on the EOL was an effect of group present, $\chi^2(2, N = 109) = 16.17, p < .001$. Planned comparisons revealed that controls responded "not sure" more often than the mild TBI group, $\chi^2(1, N = 72) = 13.45, p < .001$, and more often than the severe TBI group, $\chi^2(1, N = 69) = 10.55, p < .002$, but the severe and mild groups did not differ significantly from one another. We found that for each of the three judgments there was a strong effect of age at test on confidence, with older children more likely to choose the "not sure" judgment than younger children, $\chi^2(1, N = 109) = 4.03, p < .05$.

Correlation between EOL judgment and measure of learning.   Of practical interest is the extent to which accuracy of metacognitive judgments can influence learning. In other words, are children who are more accurate in their metacognitive judgments also better learners? To address this issue, we looked at the correlation between accuracy of EOL judgments and the degree of learning displayed for each participant. Across all participants, the correlation between EOL accuracy and degree of learning as measured by the increase in words recalled from Trial 1 to Trial 3 was $r = .28$. Though this is not a high correlation, it was statistically significant, $p = .04$. Thus it appears that there is at least a weak relation between the ability to judge the difficulty in learning an item and the subsequent ability to learn that item.

In summary, children with severe head injury were impaired relative to typically developing control children on metacognitive judgments that involved making predictions for performance on individual items (EOL judgments). Given experience with the items, their ability to make predictions about later recall of the items (JOL) did not differ significantly from the controls, nor did the ability to retrospectively evaluate their performance immediately after recall (JOK). Children with TBI overestimated their abilities to a greater degree than did control children, and were more confident in their judgments. There was a nonsignificant trend for children with severe TBI to learn less over trials than control children, but no differences in the measure of forgetting after delay. Finally, across all participants, better performance on the EOL judgment was weakly, but significantly, correlated with better recall performance. There was also a general effect of age at test, with older children in each group performing better than younger children.

METACOGNITION AND LANGUAGE PROCESSING

Sentence Anomaly Detection and Repair (Dennis et al., 1996; Martin & Romani, 1994)

It has been suggested that metacognition plays a part in language processing in the analysis of metalinguistic knowledge in the form of tacit understanding of grammatical structure as well as pragmatic rules (Dennis et al., 1996; Sutter & Johnson, 1990). Furthermore, the link between working memory and comprehension has been hypothesized to be mediated by metacognitive abilities (Swanson & Trahan, 1996). To investigate metacognition and working memory within the language comprehension domain we utilized an auditory sentence anomaly detection and repair task in which children were asked to make acceptability judgments for sentences that did or did not contain a semantic anomaly. Once the anomaly was detected, it was to be explicitly identified by the participant and finally, the participant was asked to repair the anomaly.

Method

Participants.   We tested 36 children with severe, nonpenetrating TBI score (GCS = 3–8), 52 children with mild TBI (GCS = 13–15), and 44 typically developing children (Controls). Table 2 shows age, gender, and injury characteristics for each group. Age at test was included as a covariate. Preliminary analyses indicated that the three groups did not differ significantly on age at test ($p = .53$) and had similar distributions. Neither age at injury ($p = .88$) nor interval since injury ($p = 12$) varied significantly between the mild and severe groups.

TABLE 2
Age and Injury Characteristics of Children in the Control, Mild TBI, and Severe TBI Groups for the Sentence Anomaly Detection Task

Group (n)	Mean Age-at-Test in Years (Range)	Mean Age-at-Injury in Years (Range)	Mean Interval Since Injury in Years (Range)	GCS Mean (SD)	Boys (no.)/ Girls (no.)
Control (44)	12.1 (5.3–16.7)	na	na	na	17/15
Mild TBI (52)	12.1 (5.1–16.4)	6.7 (0.6–12.1)	5.4 (2.1–14.9)	14.6 (.69)	26/14
Severe TBI (36)	11.5 (6.7–14.8)	6.8 (1.1–11.9)	4.9 (1.9–11.1)	7.6 (2.8)	23/14

Note.   TBI = traumatic brain injury: GCS = Glasgow Coma Scale.

Materials and procedure.   A set of 24 sentences was constructed such that 12 were sensible (acceptable) sentences, and 12 contained anomalies that were violations of a semantic or pragmatic rule ("She threw the fried boots in the garbage"). In addition, memory load was varied within sentences so that half the sentences in each condition were high memory load, and half were low memory load (Hanten et al., 1999). The child was instructed to listen to each sentence carefully, and to press a key just as soon as he or she knew whether a sentence was acceptable or unacceptable. If the sentence was a "good" sentence, the child pressed a computer key marked with green tape, but if the sentence was bad, the child pressed a different key labeled with red tape. If the child correctly indicated that the sentence was unacceptable, then she or he was asked to identify the anomaly, and then to provide a repair for the correctly identified anomaly. Measures include the percentage of correct acceptability responses to the sentences (anomaly detection), the percentage of detected anomalies that were correctly identified, and a repair score. The repair score was calculated so that children received 2 points for correctly and specifically repairing the anomaly and preserving the meaning of the whole sentence, and 1 point was given for producing a sentence that was correct, but did not preserve the meaning of the original sentence. The child was required to respond to the acceptability portion of the task after hearing the sentence only once. However, once the child decided that the sentence was anomalous, she or he was allowed to hear the sentence again, if requested, to perform the identification and repair portions of the task. The total testing time for this task was approximately 20 min.

Data analysis: As in the previous experiment, we modeled the outcome with severity group, using age at test as a covariate, by generalized estimating equation (GEE) model. The SAS procedure GENMOD and logit or log link function was used depending on the form of the outcome variables. The GENMOD procedure fits a GEE model to the data by maximum likelihood estimation of the parameter vectors, the statistic of interest being Likelihood Ratio chi-square.

Results

Two sets of analyses were done for this experiment. The first set compared performance in the TBI groups to that in the noninjured control group for detecting anomalous sentences or accepting sensible sentences, for identifying anomalies in sentences in which anomalies were detected, and for repairing identified anomalies. In the sentence anomaly experiment, a repeated measures model was fitted with group (Mild TBI, Severe TBI, or Control), age at test and their interactions as a between-subject factors, and sentence type (Sensible or Anomalous) as within-subject factors. A separate analysis was done with memory load (High or Low) as the within-subject factor.

Anomaly Detection Data

Repeated measures analysis of anomaly detection data revealed significant main effects of (a) group, $\chi^2(2, N = 132) = 5.87$, $p = .05$, and (b) sentence type, $\chi^2(1, N = 132) = 8.64$, $p < .01$, with responses to sensible sentences more accurate than to anomalous sentences. There was an interaction of group with sentence type, $\chi^2(2, N = 132) = 8.07$, $p = .01$, indicating that on the anomalous sentences the uninjured children were significantly more accurate than either the mild, $\chi^2(1, N = 96) = 4.89$, $p < .05$, or the severe TBI group, $\chi^2(1, N = 80) = 11.15$, $p < .01$. On the sensible sentences the groups did not differ significantly from each other. Figure 5 shows the least square means of correct judgments by sentence type and group. Younger children made more errors than did older children, $\chi^2(1, N = 132) = 22.08$, $p < .01$. There was no interaction of age at test with group.

Anomaly identification data.   There were no significant differences in the ability to specifically identify anomalies in correctly rejected anomalous sentences.

Anomaly repair data.   There was no significant effect of injury severity on the ability to provide an adequate repair of anomalous sentences. As with the

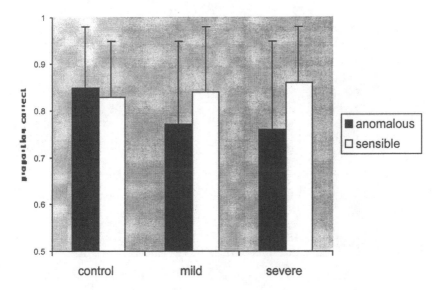

FIGURE 5   Proportion correct judgments (bars = *SD*) for anomalous and sensible sentences by head injury group.

anomaly detection, there was a large effect of age at test, $\chi^2(1, N = 132) = 169.73, p$ < .0001, but no interaction.

Working memory and anomaly detection.   A separate analysis of the effect of memory load on anomaly detection replicated the overall effect of injury severity, $\chi^2(2, N = 132) = 5.86, p < .05$, and revealed a main effect of working memory load on anomaly detection, with a significant advantage of sentences with low memory load over those with high memory load, $\chi^2(1, N = 132) = 5.32, p < .05$. Planned comparisons indicated that the three groups did not differ significantly on the low memory load sentences, but on the high memory load sentences, the children with severe TBI performed significantly worse than the control children, $\chi^2(1, N = 80) = 4.18, p < .05$. The mild TBI group and the control group did not differ significantly from each other. Figure 6 shows the correct judgments on anomaly detection by group and memory load condition. Younger children performed significantly more poorly than did older children, $\chi^2(1, N = 132) = 22.20, p < .01$, but there was no interaction of age at test with injury severity.

Summary of Sentence Anomaly Detection and Repair Task

Children with severe and mild TBI were impaired relative to typically developing control children on their ability to detect semantic anomalies within spoken sen-

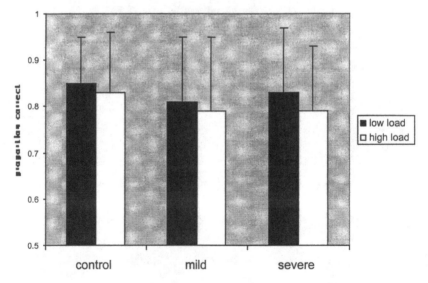

FIGURE 6   Proportion correct judgments (bars = *SD*) for anomaly detection task by head injury group and memory load condition.

tences. The children with severe TBI were particularly impaired on sentences with a high memory load. There were no group differences in the ability to repair detected anomalies. There was an overall effect of age at test, with younger children performing more poorly than older children.

GENERAL DISCUSSION

The data presented here are consistent with an interpretation of impaired executive-level functioning in metacognition, as a consequence of childhood severe TBI. We have shown that metacognitive deficits are evident in children with TBI, and, further, that different forms of metacognition bear different relations to core cognitive domains such as memory and language.

Within the memory domain, children with severe TBI were impaired relative to children with mild TBI and uninjured children in their ability to accurately predict the ease of learning of specific items within a list-learning task. Performance on this judgment approximated chance. In contrast, after gaining experience with the stimulus items, children with TBI were as able as uninjured children in monitoring their degree of learning, though the level of accuracy still remained rather low (.59 of the words were accurately predicted). Finally, when retrospectively assessing their performance on recall, children of all groups were quite accurate, with over .90 of the words correctly predicted across groups, with no significant differences among the groups.

It has been previously reported that under conditions of item-by-item judgments, typically developing children, as well as adults, tend to overestimate their abilities to a considerable degree (Schneider et al., 2000). We found that children with TBI had an exaggerated effect of overestimation of memory span based on the EOL. The findings of impairment with the EOL judgment, but not with the other two judgments, taken with the exaggerated overestimation of memory span, suggests that the metacognitive monitoring deficit observed may be the consequence of a failure to adequately integrate metacognitive self knowledge with metacognitive monitoring abilities. In the EOL judgment, children had to prospectively assess their own memory span and relate that to item-by-item judgments to come up with an accurate estimation of ease of learning. In the two judgments (JOL and JOK) following the study and test trials, the participants would retrospectively monitor their performance and make a prediction presumably based on their past performance over trials, thus it is reasonable to postulate that memory for their past performance, which in this study did not differ among groups, may be a contributing factor in the JOL and JOK measures. Only in the EOL judgment was the child called on to make a judgment based solely on self-knowledge and projection.

Consistent with the overestimation of memory span, children with TBI were less likely than control children to be uncertain of their performance, regardless of actual performance. This suggests that children who have sustained TBI may display deficits in metacognitive abilities, especially those relating to self-knowledge of abilities.

Children show verbal memory and learning deficits after severe TBI (Anderson, Catroppa, Rosenfeld, Haritou, & Morse, 2000; Levin, 1989; Levin, Eisenberg, Wiggs, & Kobayashi, 1982; Levin et al., 1988; Yeates, Blumenstein, Patterson, & Delis, 1995). These results, however, cannot be accounted for by differences in memory span because groups did not differ in recall trials. It may be that forms of executive memory less studied in TBI populations, such as working memory and prospective memory, are more important than declarative memory for successful metacognition. The relation between executive memory and metacognition would be a fruitful area to explore.

Even regarding standard verbal learning tasks, the procedural implementation for the study–recall trials in this study varies from that of other verbal learning tests in several important ways. The items in our lists were abstract words, with minimal semantic relations among the items. When prevented from using semantic strategies, as in the case of recall of abstract words, control children and children with mild TBI might be expected to perform at a level more similar to children with severe TBI. This is consistent with reports of adult patients' failure to use semantic information as an aid in recall (Levin & Goldstein, 1986).

Presentation mode may also be relevant, which here was single-presentation visual rather than paced and verbal. Visual presentation may provide a recall advantage for adult patients with auditory–verbal short-term memory deficits (Shallice & Vallar, 1990) and for children with TBI who have verbal learning deficits (Hanten & Martin, 2000). The longer presentation time may interact with the modality factor and allow for compensation for effects of slowed processing speed that may be present among the TBI patients.

The data on language monitoring support the view that impairments in metacognition are accounted for by deficits in executive memory rather than in traditional declarative memory and learning. Here, working memory proved to be important.

All children performed better on sensible than on anomalous sentences. This effect was not due to an "accept" response bias nor poor attentional abilities because anomalous sentences with a greater memory load were responded to more poorly than were anomalous sentences with a lesser memory load; both a bias response account or an attentional account of our findings requires a uniform response across memory load conditions, which did not occur. Importantly, children with severe TBI were impaired relative to children with mild TBI and control children in the ability to monitor spoken language to detect semantic anomalies. The effect was greater for sentences with high working memory requirement, and there was a pronounced effect of age at test.

Children with TBI have difficulty detecting sentence anomaly (Dennis et al., 1996). These results extend this finding by showing further that working memory contributed to the difficulty of children who have sustained severe TBI in detecting anomalies in spoken sentences. Whereas, in our preliminary study of the performance of children with severe TBI on the sentence anomaly detection task (Hanten et al., 1999), we found that children with severe TBI were impaired relative to uninjured children on the specific identification of anomalies, in the repair of anomalous sentences, in this expanded study, in agreement with Dennis et al. (1996) we found no such effect. Within the language domain, deficits in language monitoring are not inevitably accompanied by deficits in metalinguistic knowledge.

Age at test emerged as a significant factor in performance for most of the measures employed in this study. The notable exceptions were the measure of metacognitive monitoring in the memory domain (i.e., the EOL, JOL, and JOK). There is a vast literature detailing the developmental increases in memory abilities, much of which focuses on the concurrent increases in memory span and metacognitive functioning. In our study, we found age at test effects in the acquisition of metacognitive knowledge (as measured by self-knowledge of memory span and in overconfidence in judgments) and, correspondingly, the expected age-related increases in recall. However, metacognitive monitoring did not seem to be moderated by age in the memory domain. In contrast, monitoring within the language domain was strongly affected by age. These data underscore the importance of normative data on typically developing children in studies of complex cognitive functions with a protracted developmental course.

Severity of injury, as measured by GCS score, had a moderating effect on many of the measures. For most measures, children with severe TBI performed significantly worse than either the children with mild TBI or the typically developing children on measures of metacognitive ability.

Metacognition is considered to be an executive function, and, as such, is affected by the integrity of the frontal lobes. Brain imaging studies of the neuropathology of nonpenetrating TBI have demonstrated that the prefrontal region of persons with severe TBI is often selectively damaged by structural (Levin et al., 1997) and functional (Langfitt et al., 1986) lesions. Regardless of the location of the original impact, TBI appears to be characterized by diffuse generalized damage with superimposed focal damage to frontal polar and anterior temporal areas (Adams, 1975). PET scanning studies of persons with severe TBI have documented that cerebral hypometabolism is a frequent sequel, which typically involves or is focused in the prefrontal region (Langfitt et al., 1986). The areas of cortex most predisposed to contusion are the frontal poles, the orbital gyri cortex adjacent to the Sylvian fissure, and the inferior and lateral surfaces of the temporal lobes. This characteristic distribution of contusion has been interpreted to be the result of the proximity of these areas to the sphenoidal ridges and bony pro-trusions on the base of the skull (Adams, 1975; Bigler, 1990). Thus, it appears that frontal lobe damage and resulting impairments of executive functioning are likely consequences of TBI. The data presented here adds to the growing body of evidence that children, as well as adults, experience deficits in executive functioning, and specifically in metacognition, as a consequence of severe TBI. The particular neuropathology patterns involved in these deficits remain to be elucidated.

In summary, we have described deficits of metacognitive monitoring, within the memory domain in prospective, but not retrospective, judgments of recall (EOL), and, within the language domain, impairments of monitoring of spoken language for semantic content. Metacognitive knowledge impairment for memorial abilities was demonstrated in children with severe TBI by poor estimation of memory span and exaggerated overconfidence in performance, but in the language domain, metalinguistic knowledge in the form of adequate repairs of anomalous sentences was preserved. The findings of small differences between the children with TBI and the uninjured control children on measures of learning and forgetting in the memory task, as well as the effects of working memory load in the sentence processing task, hint that metacognitive control may also be impaired, though further research is needed.

ACKNOWLEDGMENTS

This work was supported in part by Grant NS21889 from the National Institutes of Health.

REFERENCES

Adams, J. H. (1975). The neuropathology of head injury. In P. J. Vinken & G. W. Bruyn (Eds.), *Handbook of clinical neurology* (Vol. 23, pp. 35–65). New York: Elsevier.

Anderson, V. A., Catroppa, C., Rosenfeld, J., Haritou, F., & Morse, S. (2000). Recovery of memory function following traumatic brain injury in pre-school children. *Brain Injury, 14,* 679–692.

Appel, L. F., Cooper, R. B., McCarrell, N., Sims-Knight, J., Yussen, S., & Flavell, J. H. (1972). The development of the distinction between perceiving and memorizing. *Child Development, 43,* 1365–1381.

Bigler, E. D. (1990). Neuropathology of traumatic brain injury. In E. D. Bigler (Ed.), *Traumatic brain injury* (pp. 13–49). Austin, TX: PRO-ED.

Brown, A. L. (1978). Knowing when, where, and how to remember: A problem of metacognition. In R. Glaser (Ed.), *Advances in instructional psychology* (pp. 367–406). Hillsdale, NJ: Lawrence Erlbaum Associates, Inc.

Brown, A. L., & DeLoache, J. S. (1978). Skills, plans, and self-regulation. In R. S. Siegler (Ed.), *Children's thinking: What develops?* (pp. 3–35). Hillsdale, NJ: Lawrence Erlbaum Associates, Inc.

Chapman, S., Watkins, R., Gustafson, C., Moore, S., Levin, H. S., & Kufera, J. A. (1997). Narrative discourse in children with closed head injury, children with language impairment, and typically developing children. *American Journal of Speech and Language Pathology, 6,* 66–75.

Dennis, M., Barnes, M. A., Donnelly, R. E., Wilkinson, M., & Humphreys, R. (1996). Appraising and managing knowledge: Metacognitive skills after childhood head injury. *Developmental Neuropsychology, 12,* 17–34.

Dennis, M., Wilkinson, M., Koski, L., & Humphreys, R. P. (1995). Attention deficits in the long term after childhood head injury. In S. H. Broman & M. E. Michel (Eds.), *Traumatic head injury in children* (pp. 165–187). New York: Oxford University Press.

Dufresne, A., & Kobasigawa, A. (1989). Children's spontaneous allocation of study times: Differential and sufficient aspects. *Journal of Experimental Child Psychology, 47,* 274–296.

Ewing-Cobbs, L., Prasad, M., Fletcher, J. M., Levin, H. S., Miner, M. E., & Eisenberg, H. M. (1998). Attention after pediatric traumatic brain injury: A multidimensional assessment. *Child Neuropsychology, 4,* 35–48.

Flavell, J. H., Beach, D. R., & Chinsky, J. M. (1966). Spontaneous verbal rehearsal in a memory task as a function of age. *Child Development, 37,* 283–299.

Flavell, J. H., Friedrichs, A., & Hoyt, J. (1970). Developmental changes in memorization processes. *Cognitive Psychology, 1,* 324–340.

Flavell, J. H., Green, F. L., & Flavell, E. R. (1985). The road not taken: Understanding the implications of initial uncertainty in evaluating spatial directions. *Developmental Psychology, 21,* 207–216.

Garrity, L. I. (1975). An electronmyographical study of subvocal speech and recall in preschool children. *Developmental Psychology, 11,* 274–281.

Hanten, G., Bartha, M., & Levin, H. S. (2000). Metacognition following pediatric traumatic brain injury: A preliminary study. *Developmental Neuropsychology, 18,* 383–398.

Hanten, G., Levin, H. S., & Song, J. X. (1999). Working memory and metacognition in sentence comprehension by severely head-injured children: A preliminary study. *Developmental Neuropsychology, 16,* 393–414.

Hanten, G., & Martin, R. C. (2000). Contributions of phonological and semantic short-term memory to sentence processing: Evidence from two cases of closed head injury in children. *Journal of Memory & Language, 43,* 335–361.

Holcomb, P., Coffey, S., & Neville, H. (1992). Visual and auditory sentence processing: A developmental analysis using event-related brain potentials. *Developmental Neuropsychology, 8,* 203–241.

Keeney, T. J., Cannizzo, S. R., & Flavell, J. H. (1967). Spontaneous and induced verbal rehearsal in a recall task. *Child Development, 38,* 953–966.

Kennedy, B. A., & Miller, D. J. (1976). Persistent use of verbal rehearsal as a function of information about its value. *Child Development, 47,* 566–569.

Langfitt, T. W., Obrist, W. D., Alavi, A., Grossman, R. I., Zimmerman, R., Jaggi, J., et al. (1986). Computerized tomography, magnetic resonance imaging and positron emission tomography in the study of brain trauma. Preliminary observations. *Journal of Neurosurgery, 64,* 760–767.

Leonesio, R. J., & Nelson, T. O. (1990). Do different metamemory judgments tap the same underlying aspects of memory? *Journal of Experimental Psychology, 16,* 464–470.

Levin, H. S. (1989). Memory deficit after closed head injury. *Journal of Clinical and Experimental Neuropsychology, 12,* 129–153.

Levin, H. S., Eisenberg, H. M., Wiggs, C. L., & Kobayashi, K. (1982). Memory and intellectual ability after head injury in children and adolescents. *Neurosurgery, 11,* 668–673.

Levin, H. S., Fletcher, J. M., Kufera, J. A., Harward, H., Lilly, M., Mendelsohn, D., et al. (1996). Dimensions of cognition measured by the Tower of London and other cognitive tasks in head injured children and adolescents. *Developmental Neuropsychology, 12,* 17–34.

Levin, H. S., & Goldstein, F. C. (1986). Organization of verbal memory after severe closed-head injury. *Journal of Clinical and Experimental Neuropsychology, 8,* 643–656.

Levin, H. S., High, W. H., Ewing-Cobbs, L., Fletcher, J. M., Eisenberg, H. M., Miner, M. E., et al. (1988). Memory functioning during the first year after closed-head injury in children and adolescents. *Neurosurgery, 22,* 1043–1052.

Levin, H. S., Mendelsohn, D., Lilly, M., Yeakley, J., Song, J. X., Scheibel, R. S., et al. (1997). Magnetic resonance imaging in relation to functional outcome of pediatric closed head injury: A test of the Ommaya-Gennarelli model. *Neurosurgery, 40,* 432–440.

Liu, H., Bates, E., Powell, T., & Wulfeck, B. (1997). Single word shadowing and the study of lexical access. *Applied Psycholinguistics, 18,* 157–180.

Martin, R. C., & Romani, C. (1994). Verbal working memory and sentence comprehension. A multi-component view. *Neuropsychology, 8,* 506–523.

Mazzoni, G., & Nelson, T. O. (Eds.). (1998). *Metacognition and cognitive neuropsychology: Monitoring and control processes.* Mahwah, NJ: Lawrence Erlbaum Associates, Inc.

Metcalfe, J., & Shimamura, A. P. (1994). *Metacognition: Knowing about knowing.* Cambridge, MA: MIT.

Moynahan, E. D. (1973). The development of knowledge concerning the effect of categorization upon free recall. *Child Development, 44,* 238–246.

Nelson, T. O. (Ed.). (1992). *Metacognition: Core readings.* Boston: Allyn & Bacon.

Rogoff, B., Newcombe, N. E., & Kagan, J. (1974). The development of knowledge concerning the effect of categorization upon free recall. *Child Development, 44,* 238–236.

Schneider, W. (1998). The development of procedural metamemory in childhood and adolescence. In G. Mazzoni & T. O. Nelson (Eds.), *Metacognition and cognitive neuropsychology: Monitoring and control processes* (pp. 1–21). Mahwah, NJ: Lawrence Erlbaum Associates, Inc.

Schneider, W., Visé, M., Lockl, K., & Nelson, T. O. (2000). Developmental trends in children's memory monitoring: Evidence from a judgment-of-learning task. *Cognitive Development, 15,* 115–134.

Shallice, T., & Vallar, G. (1990). The impairment of auditory-verbal short-term storage. In V. G. & T. Shallice (Eds.), *Neuropsychological impairments of short-term memory* (pp. 11–53). Cambridge, England: Cambridge University Press.

Sutter, J. C., & Johnson, C. J. (1990). School-aged children's metalinguistic awareness of grammaticality in verb form. *Journal of Speech and Hearing Research, 33,* 84–95.

Swanson, H. L., & Trahan, M. (1996). Learning disabled and average reader's working memory and comprehension: Does metacognition play a role? *British Journal of Educational Psychology, 66,* 333–355.

Teasdale, G., & Jennett, B. (1974). Assessment of coma and impaired consciousness: A practical scale. *Lancet, 2,* 81–84.

Tyler, L. K., & Marlsen-Wilson, W. D. (1981). Children's processing of spoken language. *Journal of Verbal Learning and Verbal Behavior, 20,* 400–416.

Wellman, H. M., Collins, J., & Glieberman, J. (1981). Understanding the combination of memory variables: Developing conceptions of memory limitations. *Child Development, 52,* 1313–1317.

Worden, P. E., & Sladewski-Awig, L. J. (1982). Children's awareness of memorability. *Journal of Educational Psychology, 74,* 341–350.

Yeates, K. O., Blumenstein, E., Patterson, C. M., & Delis, D. C. (1995). Verbal learning and memory following pediatric closed-head injury. *Journal of the International Neuropsychological Society, 1,* 78–87.

DEVELOPMENTAL NEUROPSYCHOLOGY, 25(1&2), 107–133
Copyright © 2004, Lawrence Erlbaum Associates, Inc.

Modeling of Longitudinal Academic Achievement Scores After Pediatric Traumatic Brain Injury

Linda Ewing-Cobbs

Department of Pediatrics
University of Texas Houston Health Science Center

Marcia Barnes

Department of Psychology
Hospital for Sick Children
Toronto, Ontario, Canada

Jack M. Fletcher

Department of Pediatrics
University of Texas Houston Health Science Center

Harvey S. Levin

Cognitive Neuroscience Laboratory
Departments of Physical Medicine and Rehabilitation, Neurosurgery, and
Psychiatry and Behavioral Sciences
Baylor College of Medicine
Houston, TX

Paul R. Swank

Department of Pediatrics
University of Texas Houston Health Science Center

James Song

Department of Biometry
Bayer Pharmaceuticals
New Haven, CT

Requests for reprints should be sent to Linda Ewing-Cobbs, Department of Pediatrics, University of Texas Houston Health Science Center, Houston, TX 77030. E-mail: linda.ewing-cobbs@uth.tmc.edu

In a prospective longitudinal study, academic achievement scores were obtained from youth 5 to 15 years of age who sustained mild–moderate ($n = 34$) or severe ($n = 43$) traumatic brain injuries (TBI). Achievement scores were collected from baseline to 5 years following TBI and were subjected to individual growth curve analysis. The models fitted age at injury, years since injury, duration of impaired consciousness, and interaction effects to Reading Decoding, Reading Comprehension, Spelling, and Arithmetic standard scores. Although scores improved significantly over the follow-up relative to normative data from the standardization sample of the tests, children with severe TBI showed persistent deficits on all achievement scores in comparison to children with mild–moderate TBI. Interactions of the slope and age parameters for the Arithmetic and Reading Decoding scores indicated greater increases over time in achievement scores of the children injured at an older age, but deceleration in growth curves for the younger children with both mild–moderate and severe TBI. These results are compatible with the hypothesis that early brain injuries disrupt the acquisition of some academic skills. Hierarchical regression models revealed that indexes of academic achievement obtained 2 years following TBI had weak relations with the duration of impaired consciousness and socioeconomic status. In contrast, concurrent cognitive variables such as phonological processing and verbal memory accounted for more variability in academic scores. Given the significant and persistent decrement in basic academic skills in youth with severe TBI, it is clear that head-injured youth require intensive, long-term remediation and intervention not only of the academic skills themselves, but also of those cognitive abilities that support the development and maintenance of reading and math.

Success in school settings is essential for educational attainment, psychosocial adjustment, and eventual vocational adaptation (Rivera-Batz, 1992; Spreen, 1988). Despite the knowledge that children who have sustained traumatic brain injury (TBI) experience a significant degree of academic failure, there has been limited characterization of dimensions of academic achievement in children and adolescents with TBI. Understanding the academic difficulties experienced by students after TBI is important for developing appropriate interventions and in maximizing long-term adjustment. To understand the nature of academic difficulties experienced by youth with TBI, it is necessary to investigate the developmental course of growth and recovery of academic skills after TBI as well as those variables that predict growth and recovery. This is particularly relevant given that academic scores often recover to the average range in school-aged children and adolescents after moderate to severe TBI, but these average scores are not paralleled by comparable average academic performance (Ewing-Cobbs, Fletcher, Levin, Iovino, & Miner, 1998). This article presents a longitudinal study of the development of reading decoding, reading comprehension, spelling, and arithmetic skills in youth after mild–moderate and severe TBI in which injury-related variables (duration of impaired consciousness), developmental variables (age at injury, time since injury), environmental variables (e.g., socioeconomic status), and concurrent cognitive variables (e.g., memory, vocabulary knowledge) are used to model academic achievement.

INJURY SEVERITY AND RELATION TO ACADEMIC ACHIEVEMENT AND FUNCTIONAL ACADEMIC OUTCOME

Longitudinal and cross-sectional studies evaluating academic achievement scores and academic performance after pediatric TBI indicated that academic variables were significantly related to the severity of brain injury (Barnes, Dennis, & Wilkinson, 1999; Chadwick, Rutter, Shaffer, & Shrout, 1981; Ewing-Cobbs et al., 1998; Fay, Jaffe, Polissar, Liao, Rivara, & Martin, 1994). When scores are adjusted for prior risk factors, mild TBI does not appear to be associated with a significant decrease in math, spelling, or reading scores (Bijur, Haslum, & Golding, 1990; Fay et al., 1993). At 1 year after TBI, Jaffe and colleagues (1993) determined that injury severity was associated with the largest and most consistent deficits on academic achievement and intelligence tests in comparison to other neuropsychological measures. Children with severe TBI have scored lower than either children with mild injuries or community controls on a variety of achievement scores during the early stages of recovery as well as 6 months to several years after the injury (Barnes et al., 1999; Chadwick et al., 1981; Ewing-Cobbs et al., 1998; Jaffe et al., 1992; Jaffe et al., 1993; Knights et al., 1991). However, Kinsella et al. (1995) did not identify significant differences in academic achievement scores in children with varying injury severities at either 3- or 12-month follow-up intervals. The difference in findings across studies may be related to the relatively small sample and few children with severe TBI in the group described by Kinsella and colleagues.

The pattern of academic skill deficits is uneven in children after TBI. Studies comparing Wide Range Achievement Test (Jastak & Jastak, 1978) scores in different content areas revealed that word recognition scores were relatively spared, whereas arithmetic scores were the most vulnerable to disruption by TBI (Berger-Gross & Shackelford, 1985; Ewing-Cobbs et al., 1998; Levin & Benton, 1985). The sensitivity of the arithmetic subtest may be due in part to the demands of the task for both speed and power; the word recognition and spelling subtests are untimed. The few studies assessing reading comprehension suggested mild reduction in scores related to the severity of injury (Barnes et al., 1999; Ewing-Cobbs et al., 1998).

After childhood TBI, achievement test scores suggest generally good recovery of basic academic achievement skills. In contrast, several indexes of academic performance or functional academic outcome indicate persistent deficits. Ewing-Cobbs and colleagues (1998) followed children and adolescents for 2 years after mild–moderate and severe TBI; only 21% of severely injured children and adolescents were promoted each year and received a regular educational curriculum despite generally average achievement scores. Children with severe TBI were significantly more likely to receive special educational services than children with milder injuries 1 to 2 years after the injury (Donders, 1994; Ewing-Cobbs et al., 1998; Kinsella et al., 1995; Kinsella et al., 1997). Comparison of group administered academic achievement test scores from school records revealed significant declines in reading and language areas from 1 to 2 years prior to the injury to 3 years after TBI (Stallings, Ewing-Cobbs, Francis, & Fletcher, 1995). Other indexes of academic performance, such as classroom grades, declined in severely injured children relative to children with lesser injuries (Fay et al., 1994). These findings underscore the dissociation between academic competence and academic performance. Although most children master basic academic skills following TBI, they have marked difficulties using these skills competently in academic settings.

Because academic achievement scores do not adequately characterize the academic difficulties that youth with TBI experience in the classroom setting, it is important to expand assessment of academic skills to include a broader range of academic variables. Assessment of academic competence should include indexes of the child's performance in the classroom, including measures of the adequacy of task initiation and completion, difficulties in abstraction, dysregulation of attention and behavior, decreases in the rate of learning new information, disruption of metacognitive processes, and difficulty producing and processing oral and written discourse (Ewing-Cobbs & Bloom, 2004). Parent and teacher ratings of children's academic performance also suggest significant academic deficits following severe TBI. Parent and teacher ratings of children's academic performance on the Child Behavior Checklist and Teacher's Report Form (Achenbach, 1991) indicated significant declines from preinjury academic performance after severe TBI (Fay et al., 1993; Rivara et al., 1994; Taylor, Yeates, Wade, Drotar, & Klein, 1999). Children with severe TBI had significantly reduced scores relative to children with mild to moderate TBI on the Teacher's Report Form Academic Performance variable when evaluated 1 to 4 years after TBI (Fay et al., 1993; Taylor et al., 1999). Teacher ratings may be more variable than parent ratings due to several factors, including the change in informants from year to year, and variable frames of reference for different raters (e.g., some teachers comparing children with TBI to other children receiving modified curricula and other teachers comparing to typically developing children).

RELATION OF DEVELOPMENTAL VARIABLES TO ACADEMIC ACHIEVEMENT

Age at the time of injury may be related to the severity of academic skill deficits. Children who sustained mild TBI during the preschool years had slower acquisition of reading skills by age 6.5 years than comparison children without injuries

(Wrightson, McGinn, & Gronwall, 1995). However, this study lacked a comparison group of children sustaining extracranial injury with risk factors similar to the TBI patients. In a cross-sectional study, Barnes et al. (1999) reported that children injured prior to age 6.5 years had less accurate word decoding and reading comprehension than children injured in the early primary grades. Michaud, Rivara, Jaffe, Fay, and Dailey (1993) found that head injury sustained during the preschool years significantly increased the likelihood of receipt of special educational services during elementary school. Although these studies raise important issues regarding the possible interaction of age at injury with skill development, the findings require replication with longitudinal samples, including orthopedic comparison groups to control for premorbid risk factors that predispose to injury and learning problems. Levin and Ewing-Cobbs (2001) emphasized the difficulty of dissociating the effects of TBI from preinjury risk factors in infants and preschool-aged children as well as in children with co-morbid disorders. For example, recent studies identified a high incidence of preinjury and secondary Attention Deficit Hyperactivity Disorder (ADHD) in samples of children and adolescents sustaining TBI (Bloom et al., 2001; Gerring et al., 1998) that may impact cognitive and behavioral measures of academic development.

Time since injury is a critically important variable for understanding the impact of TBI on subsequent development. Most studies examine recovery after TBI for about 1 year. However, the impact of TBI on the subsequent development of new skills as well as the application of previously acquired skills in novel and more complex contexts can only be evaluated using longitudinal models that characterize the developmental trajectory of different abilities over time. The few studies to examine the development of academic skills several years after moderate to severe TBI identified persisting sequelae in areas including word decoding, reading comprehension, spelling, arithmetic, and written language skills (Barnes et al., 1999; Ewing-Cobbs et al., 1998, Fay et al., 1994; Taylor et al., 2002; Wrightson et al., 1995). Word decoding appears to be an area of particular vulnerability for young children (Barnes et al., 1999; Wrightson et al., 1995).

RELATION OF ENVIRONMENTAL AND COGNITIVE VARIABLES TO ACADEMIC ACHIEVEMENT AFTER TBI

Academic achievement scores and academic performance may also be moderated by variables other than TBI severity, including socioeconomic status (SES), child and family adjustment, and gender. Less favorable outcomes after severe TBI have been associated with lower SES, poor preinjury child and family functioning, and high levels of family stress (Rivara et al., 1994; Taylor et al., 2001; Taylor et al., 1999; Yeates et al., 1997). Taylor and colleagues recently identified specific moderating effects of family variables on long-term academic performance. In youth with severe TBI, socioeconomic disadvantage was associated with declining academic performance; high levels of family stress adversely affected development of mathematical competence (Taylor et al., 2002).

In addition to indexes of injury severity and family environment, measures of other cognitive skills that are functionally related to academic skill development may also predict academic performance following pediatric TBI. Kinsella et al. (1997) examined early and concurrent neuropsychological predictors of special education placement 2 years after TBI. After adjusting for injury severity using the Glasgow Coma Scale score, only verbal learning and memory test scores obtained 3 months after TBI contributed to prediction of class placement at 2 years after TBI. When concurrent neuropsychological predictors and Wide Range Achievement Test (WRAT)–R scores were examined, none contributed to prediction of special education placement after controlling for injury severity.

Cognitive variables that are predictive of achievement scores in typically developing children and in children with learning disabilities may also predict performance in children with TBI. The normal acquisition of reading decoding is related to a small set of developmental precursors including: (a) phonological awareness, the ability to hear and manipulate the individual sounds or units of sound in words; (b) rapid visual naming of objects, letters, and colours, which is thought to be particularly related to later deficits in reading rate; and (c) print awareness, which includes knowledge about the functions of print, as well as the ability to recognize letters of the alphabet (Adams, 1991; Morris et al., 1998; Wagner, Torgesen, & Rashotte, 1994; Wolf & Bowers, 1999). Reading comprehension is highly related to both accuracy and fluency in word decoding, but also to the integrity of general language comprehension and comprehension-related skills (Gough, Hoover, & Peterson, 1996), such as vocabulary knowledge, syntactic processing, verbal working memory, and inferential comprehension (Gottardo, Stanovich, & Siegel, 1996). In children with TBI, reading fluency has been shown to be deficient and predictive of reading comprehension (Barnes et al., 1999), and difficulties with listening comprehension skills such as inferencing are also apparent (Barnes & Dennis, 2001). Spelling competence has been related to phonological processing, orthographic processing, and visual matching (Lennox & Siegel, 1996). Additionally, children with low scores on spelling and arithmetic tasks showed disruption in visual memory (Fletcher, 1985) as well as graphomotor skills required for production of written text (van der Vlugt & Satz, 1985). Because fine motor and visual motor skills are frequently disrupted in children with TBI (Thompson et al., 1994), written spelling may be related to visual motor competence. Difficulties in arithmetic calculation have been hypothesized to be related to problems in the retrieval of math facts from memory, which might depend on adequate verbal working memory; problems in learning computational strategies and procedures; and difficulties in the spatial manipulation and representation of numerical information (Geary, 1993; McLean & Hitch, 1992; Rourke, 1993). In contrast to reading, very little is known about arithmetic skill after pediatric TBI, particularly regarding whether the cognitive abilities that are related to arithmetic competence in normally developing and learning disabled children are also related to computational skill in children with TBI.

In addition to the level of basic academic skills, academic performance in the classroom is strongly related to the development of self-management skills (Hinshaw, 1992). For children with TBI, the relative contributions of (a) injury severity; (b) developmental variables such as age at injury; (c) environmental variables; (d) cognitive indexes of learning and memory, working memory, visual–spatial functioning, cognitive speed, and flexibility; and (e) adaptive behavioral competence to academic skill development and academic performance remain unexplored.

RESEARCH QUESTIONS AND HYPOTHESES

The purpose of this study was to evaluate change in academic achievement scores over a 5-year follow-up using growth curve modeling and to examine predictors of achievement scores 2 years after TBI. The impact of injury variables and developmental factors affecting long-term outcome after childhood TBI is best estimated based on longitudinal modeling of outcomes. Growth curve analysis allows modeling of the processes of change that underlie development and recovery of function (Fletcher, Ewing-Cobbs, Francis, & Levin, 1995). Growth curve analysis examines intraindividual change and allows characterization of the level of performance, change in performance over time, and the rate of change over time. Therefore, growth curve modeling provides a powerful approach for examining developmental changes in the rate of skill development over time as well as the interaction of variables such as age at injury with the rate of change.

For the growth curve analyses, we hypothesized that (a) children with severe TBI would show the greatest initial decline in achievement scores and the least increase over time in comparison to children with lesser injuries; (b) younger children would show greater disruption of reading recognition scores than adolescents, whereas adolescents would show greater disruption of reading comprehension scores than children; and (c) recovery would be seen in all skill areas assessed and would be best characterized as nonlinear. Regarding the predictors of academic achievement variables, we hypothesized that (d) injury severity and socioeconomic status would explain a significant proportion of variance in achievement scores and that (e) inclusion of concurrent cognitive variables in the model that were theoretically related to each achievement variable would enhance prediction of academic outcomes.

METHOD

Participants

Academic achievement scores were examined in 77 children with TBI who were evaluated on a minimum of three occasions as part of a prospective, longitudinal outcome study. Participants were recruited from Memorial Hermann Children's Hospital and John Sealy Hospital in the Houston metropolitan area. Criteria for inclusion were (a) nonmissile head injury; (b) TBI of sufficient severity to require hospitalization; (c) resolution of posttraumatic amnesia within 3 months of the injury; (d) no diagnosis of preinjury developmental disorder, including ADHD; (e) no diagnosis of learning disability resulting in provision of special education services; (f) no suspicion of physical child abuse; and (g) English as the child's primary language in the home.

Demographic and neurologic variables for study participants are provided in Table 1. Participants ranged in age from 5 to 15 years at the time of injury. Twenty-eight percent of the sample was female, $\chi^2(1, N = 77) = 0.13, p < .72$. The severity of TBI was categorized on the basis of the duration of impaired consciousness or coma duration, which was defined as the number of days that a child was unable to follow one-stage commands. Children sustaining mild to moderate TBI ($n = 34$) were unable to follow commands for less than 24 hr; severe TBI ($n = 43$) was defined as impaired consciousness persisting for at least 24 hr. The severity groups were similar in terms of demographic variables including age at injury, socioeconomic status, ethnicity, and gender (see Table 1). The lowest postresuscitation Glasgow Coma Scale (GCS) scores (Teasdale & Jennett, 1974) averaged 13.3 in the mild–moderate group and 5.7 in the severe

TABLE 1
Demographic and Neurologic Information by Severity of TBI

	Severity of TBI					
	Mild–Moderate[a]		Severe[b]		Statistics	p Value
	M	SD	M	SD		
Years at injury	9.82	3.22	9.38	3.32	$F(1, 75) = 0.35$	.56
Hollingshead Index	41.97	13.86	46.42	18.52	$F(1, 75) = 1.33$	.25
Days of coma	0.07	0.17	8.86	7.33	$F(1, 75) = 34.91$	.0001
GCS score	13.26	2.12	5.65	2.02	$F(1, 75) = 257.64$	.0001
Ethnicity (n)						
African American	31		32		$\chi^2(2) = 2.74$	.25
Anglo American	4		8			
Hispanic	0		2			

Note.   TBI = traumatic brain injury; GCS = Glasgow Coma Scale.
[a]$n = 34$. [b]$n = 43$.

TBI groups. Impaired consciousness persisted for 0.07 days in the mild–moderate group and 8.86 days in the severe TBI group.

Although age at injury was examined statistically as a continuous variable, age was treated as a categorical variable with three levels (5–7, 8–11, and 12–15 years) for visual presentation of findings. The three age groups correspond to ages typically associated with (a) initial acquisition of phonological, mathematical, and orthographic symbols; (b) automatization of basic operations and development of applied reasoning skills; and (c) the consolidation of reasoning skills and application of skills to new contexts. The three age groups had comparable lowest post-resuscitation GCS scores, $F(2, 74) = p > .1$, and duration of impaired consciousness, $\chi^2(2, N = 77) = 0.10$, $p < .95$. The Hollingshead Index (Hollingshead, 1975) of socioeconomic status did not differ across the age groups, $\chi^2(8, N = 77) = 12.52$, $p < .13$.

Procedure

Each child was evaluated individually by a trained examiner in an outpatient clinic setting. As part of a battery of neuropsychological tests, participants received the WRAT (Jastak & Jastak, 1978) Reading Recognition, Spelling, and Arithmetic subtests and the Peabody Individual Achievement Test (PIAT; Dunn & Markwardt, 1970) Reading Comprehension subtest. The tests were administered in a standard order at each assessment. Achievement tests were given at baseline, 6 month, 1 year, 2 years, 3 years, 4 years, and 5 or more years postinjury. The distribution of children who received multiple evaluations was comparable for the mild–moderate and severe TBI groups, $\chi^2(4, N = 77) = 4.85$, $p < .30$. Participants received from 3 to 7 evaluations; the number in parentheses indicates the number of children receiving the specified number of assessments: 3 ($n = 11$), 4 ($n = 25$), 5 ($n = 25$), 6 ($n = 13$), and 7 ($n = 3$). This cohort of children was injured between 1983 and 1989. Although the WRAT was restandardized during this time, we chose to continue to administer the original version of the test to facilitate longitudinal analyses. To reflect the true shape of change, it is desirable to use scores that are not age-adjusted for growth curve analysis (Francis, Fletcher, Stuebing, Davidson, & Thompson, 1991). However, the WRAT has different levels for ages 5–11 and age 12 or greater; the raw scores are discontinuous across levels. Consequently, the standard scores ($M = 100$, $SD = 15$) were used in all analyses. As each Level is well standardized, it is unlikely that scores were biased when children reached age 12 and were administered Level II. The WRAT had well-established reliability and validity (Jastak & Jastak, 1978). Test–retest reliability coefficients averaged .93 across ages; test–retest reliability averaged .64 for the PIAT Reading Comprehension subtest (Dunn & Markwardt, 1970). Concurrent validity for both the WRAT and PIAT was indicated by strong relations with external academic criteria, measures of general cognitive functioning, and other achievement tests (Sattler, 1992).

Parent ratings of their child's classroom performance were based on the academic competence T score from the Child Behavior Checklist (Achenbach, 1991). This composite variable includes ratings of the child's mean performance in academic subjects, receipt of special remedial services, repetition of any grades, and the presence of academic or other school problems. To assess long-term academic performance after TBI, parent ratings were examined at the 2- and 3-year follow-up intervals. Because the Child Behavior Checklist encompasses ages 5–18, the sample size was reduced because some of the head-injured youth outgrew this age range during the follow-up. The T scores were evaluated using analysis of variance with severity of TBI as the between-subjects variable.

Statistical Analyses

Individual growth curve analyses were used to characterize the change in academic achievement scores over time. The achievement standard scores were analyzed using linear mixed models by allowing the scores to be expressed as functions of the time since the injury. Examination of the data indicated that the achievement scores were increasing over time but that the rate of increase was slowing, which represents a deceleration model. To approximate this model a three-parameter polynomial function of time was used, with intercept, slope, and curvature as the parameters. The time postinjury was centered at 1 year to minimize multicollinearity and because 1 year postinjury represents a reasonable point in time at which to compare the groups. Thus, the intercept represented the level of outcome at 1 year postinjury, the slope represented the rate of growth in the outcome at 1 year postinjury, and the curvature (quadratic term) represented the acceleration or deceleration of the curve, that is, the rate at which the slope was changing. In the first model, a random coefficients model, all of the parameters were freely estimated for each individual to determine whether the parameters had random components. Coefficients without significant random variation were then fixed for additional analyses. Once the appropriate random coefficients model was selected, we then addressed the slopes-as-outcomes model to determine which of the time-invariant covariates related to the change parameters. Included were age at injury, whether or not the child exhibited impaired consciousness for more than 24 hr, and the interactions of these terms by the slope and curvature parameters.

Because of the complexity of measuring effect sizes in growth curve models, they are reported in various ways. Cohen (1988) defines the d statistic as the difference between two means divided by the estimated standard deviation. In growth curve models, the estimated variances of slopes and intercepts are the random components of the model. Thus, slopes, intercepts, and the differences between groups on these parameters may be expressed in terms of the square root of the variances for the parameters, when those parameters are random. Second, effects can be measured in terms of the proportion of variance attributable to the effect, as in R^2. In multilevel models, of which growth curve modeling is but one example, there are two sources of variance to consider. First, there is the variance in the parameter, as mentioned earlier. Then there is also residual variance. Residual variance is the variation in the individual data points not accounted for by the model. Thus, one can express the proportion of the parameter variance accounted for by a particular effect, the proportion of the total variance, or both (parameter variance plus residual variance). We have chosen to report both.

Hierarchical linear regression was employed to examine the relations of injury severity, SES, and cognitive variables with the academic achievement scores obtained at the 2-year follow-up. For each achievement score, a model was constructed by entering the duration of impaired consciousness and SES on the first step to evaluate the contribution of injury severity and preinjury socioeconomic status to prediction of achievement scores. In step two, cognitive variables were selected from tests administered concurrently with the achievement scores to characterize the cognitive functions that were theoretically related to the level of performance of each academic measure. Due to constraints of the sample size and to maintain an appropriate subject-to-variable ratio, a maximum of three cognitive measures was included in each model.

Arithmetic scores were expected to be related to measures of working memory (Geary, 1993; McLean & Hitch, 1992), visual memory (Fletcher, 1985; Siegel & Ryan, 1989), and visual–spatial skill (Ackerman & Dykman, 1995; Rourke, 1993; Share, Moffit, & Silva, 1998). Working memory was assessed using the backward score from the Digit Span subtest (Wechsler, 1974); visual memory was estimated using the consistent long-term retrieval score from the Nonverbal Selective Reminding test (Fletcher, 1985); and visual–spatial skill was measured using the standard score from the Beery Developmental Test of Visual Motor Integration (Beery, 1982). All three measures were included in the model for Arithmetic.

Spelling scores were hypothesized to be related to phonological processing, visual memory, and visual–motor integration. These constructs were estimated using the Word Fluency standard score (Spreen & Benton, 1969), the consistent long-term retrieval score from the Nonverbal Selective Reminding test (Fletcher, 1985), and the standard score from the Beery Developmental Test of Visual Motor Integration (Beery, 1982). For the Reading Recognition subtest, Word Fluency (Spreen et al., 1969) and Rapid Automatized Naming (Denckla & Rudel, 1976) tests were included as indexes of phonological processing and fluency of retrieval of names for visual stimuli, respectively. Reading Comprehension scores were predicted using word-decoding skill measured by the Reading Recognition standard score, vocabulary knowledge measured by receptive vocabulary (Dunn & Dunn, 1981), and auditory working memory measured by the backward score from Digit Span (Wechsler, 1974).

Hypothesized predictors of the School Competence variable from the Child Behavior Checklist were (a) the Vineland Adaptive Behavior Scales composite score

(Sparrow, Balla, & Cicchetti, 1984), (b) the standard scores from the PIAT Reading Comprehension and WRAT Arithmetic subtests, and (c) the Verbal Selective Reminding continuous long-term retrieval scores as a measure of long-term verbal memory (Buschke, 1972). To control for Type I error, we held the alpha level for statistical significance at $p < .05$ for each of the five achievement outcome variables. Effect sizes are reported in terms of the R^2 for the model.

RESULTS

Growth Curve Analyses

Measures of Academic Achievement

Arithmetic.   The random coefficients model for the WRAT arithmetic score indicated that the variance for the curvature was not significant. The Akaike Information Criterion (AIC) was only marginally better (2583.6) than that for the model with the curvature term fixed (2585.5). Therefore, the curvature parameter was fixed and the model reestimated. The intercept, $Z = 5.39$, $p < .0001$, and slope, $Z = 2.96$, $p = .0015$, variance estimates were both significantly greater than zero and the AIC became substantially worse (2617.8) when the slope parameter was fixed. Thus, the model with random intercept and slope and fixed curvature was chosen for the arithmetic score. There was significant covariation between slope and intercept, $Z = -3.72$, $p = .0002$, indicating that arithmetic scores at 1 year increased at a faster rate in children with lower scores than in those with higher scores. The estimated correlation between slope and intercept was $-.74$.

Examination of the fixed components (means) indicated that the group's arithmetic level as a whole was significantly below the norm ($M = 93.0$, $SD = 9.23$), $t(76) = -6.15$, $p < .0001$, $d = .75$. The slope was significantly greater than zero, $t(76) = 3.25$, $p < .0017$, $d = .71$, indicating that the children's scores were increasing relative to the norm group at 1 year postinjury, but the curvature parameter indicated that this increase was slowing significantly over time, $t(76) = -4.94$, $p < .0001$. Because the curvature parameter was fixed, there is no variance to use for an effect size. However, we note that the change in slopes from 1 year to 2 years postinjury is 49% of the slope at 1 year.

When age at injury and coma duration were added to the model, neither variable nor their interaction was related to the curvature parameter and so these terms were dropped. In addition, the interaction of age at injury and coma duration did not relate to the slope so this term was also dropped. Finally, coma was unrelated to the rate of change in WRAT arithmetic scores so it also was dropped. The final model indicated that those in a coma for less than 24 hr had higher arithmetic scores at 1 year postinjury, $t(198) = 2.43$, $p = .0159$, $d = .71$, whereas those who were older when injured had lower scores, $t(198) = -7.51$, $p < .0001$. There was also a tendency for those who were younger at injury to have smaller differences, $t(198) = 1.72, p = .088$, between the mild–moderate and severe coma groups (see Figure 1). However, arithmetic scores increased more rapidly in youth who were older at the time of injury compared to those who were younger, $t(198) = 6.21, p < .0001$. These increases decelerated with time, $t(75) = -4.40, p < .0001$. Examining the differences in variance components between the models indicates that the covariates account for 58% of the variance in the intercepts, 75% of the variance in the slopes, and about 35% of the total variance. In fact, with age at injury and coma status controlled, the variance in slopes and the covariance between intercept and slope were no longer significant meaning that the covariates accounted for most of the consistent variation in slopes and for most of the covariation between slopes and intercepts. The intercept variance remained significant, $Z = 4.50, p < .0001$, indicating that there are other factors, unmeasured in this study, that might account for that unpredicted level variance.

Spelling. The random coefficients model for the WRAT spelling test indicated significant variance in intercepts, $Z = 5.66, p < .0001$, slopes, $Z = 3.14, p = .0008$, and the curvature term, $Z = 2.61, p = .0046$. The intercepts and slopes were not significantly related and intercepts did not relate to the curvature term, but slope and curvature were significantly related, $Z = -2.82, p = .0048$, indicating that

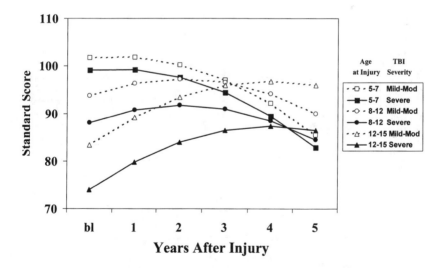

FIGURE 1   Expected values for growth curves for WRAT Arithmetic scores by severity, age, and time. Parameters for intercept and slope were significant, indicating that the severe TBI group scored lower than the mild–moderate TBI group. Although older participants had lower initial scores, their scores accelerated more over the follow-up than scores from younger participants.

those who were increasing at the faster rate relative to the norm group had rates of increase that were slowing more over time (see Figure 2).

The mean level on spelling ($M = 99.7$, $SD = 11.6$) was average and the mean rate of increase was 2.5 points per year ($SD = 4.67$, $d = .54$). The mean curvature did not differ significantly from zero. Only coma predicted level and change in spelling scores. Neither age at injury nor the interaction of age at injury with coma significantly related to intercept, slope, or curvature, so these terms were dropped from the model. Injury severity was related to the intercept in that youth with mild–moderate TBI scored on the average 8.5 points higher on spelling standard scores ($M = 104.2$) than youth with severe TBI ($M = 95.7$) at 1 year postinjury, $t(125) = 3.28$, $p = .0013$, which, based on pooled standard deviation (10.9), gives an effect size of .78. However, spelling scores increased at a faster rate in the severe group (4.1 points per year) than in the mild–moderate group (.2 points per year), $t(125) = -2.87$; $p = .0048$. Given a standard deviation of 4.3 for slopes, this reflects an effect size (d) of .91. Scores of the mild–moderate group accelerated faster than scores of the severe group, $t(125) = 2.43$, $p = .0108$. Severity as measured by length of coma accounted for 13% of the intercept variance, 16% of the slope variance, 17.4% of the curvature variance, and overall, about 11% of the total variance.

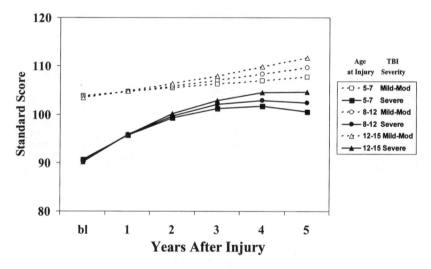

FIGURE 2   Expected values for growth curves for WRAT Spelling scores. The intercept, slope, and curvature parameters were significant. Spelling scores were lower in the severe TBI group and increased over the follow-up. Recovery curves decelerated for the severe TBI group; curves for the mild–moderate group were linear, indicating continuing improvement relative to the normative group.

Reading recognition.   A similar model was obtained for the WRAT reading scores (see Figure 3). The curvilinear term showed insignificant variance and minimal difference in the AIC from the model holding the curvature fixed. When the curvature term was fixed, the intercept had significant variance, $Z = 5.79$, $p < .0001$, as did the slope, $Z = 2.63$, $p = .0043$. The covariance between intercept and slope was not significant. The mean level at 1 year postinjury was 102.2 ($SD = 12.1$), which did not differ from 100. The fixed component of the slope was significantly greater than zero, $t(76) = 3.91$, $p = .0002$, indicating that reading standard scores were increasing 1 year postinjury at a mean rate of 2.0 points per year ($SD = 2.2$; $d = .91$). The rate of increase was slowing, however, $t(76) = -3.10$, $p = .0027$. Thus, from 1 to 2 years postinjury, we would expect slopes to decrease by about 27%.

When age at injury and coma duration were added to the model, they were unrelated to the curvature term; coma duration and the coma by age at injury interaction were unrelated to the slope; and age at injury and the age of injury by coma interaction were unrelated to the intercept. The final model indicated that coma duration was significantly related to the reading standard score at 1 year, $t(199) = 3.14$, $p = .0019$; reading recognition scores were an average of eight points higher ($SD = 11.4$) in children with mild–moderate TBI than in youth sustaining severe TBI. Severity of TBI accounted for 10.9% of the variance in intercepts. Participants in-

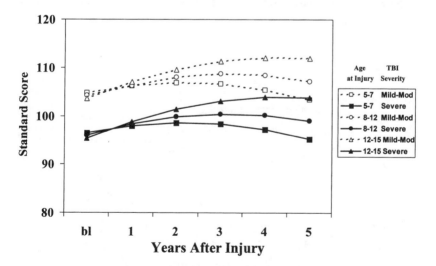

FIGURE 3   Expected values for growth curves for WRAT Reading Recognition scores. Significant variance was accounted for by the level, slope, and curvature parameters. Severe TBI was associated with lower word-decoding scores. Participants injured at an older age had greater increases in reading scores than younger participants. Although scores increased over the follow-up, the rate of change decelerated over time.

jured at a later age had greater increases in reading scores, $t(199) = 2.0, p = .0465$, but the rate of increase was declining for all respondents, $t(75) = -2.64, p = .0102$. By the 3-year follow-up, scores in both the mild–moderate and severe groups were lowest in children who were 5 to 8 years of age at the time of TBI than in older children and adolescents. Age at injury accounted for 2.5% of the variance in word-decoding slopes at 1 year postinjury. Overall, the covariates predicted 9.3% of the total variance.

Reading comprehension.   The model for reading comprehension originally included a random curvature term. However, the curvature variance was not significant and the AIC improved when the curvature term was fixed. This restricted model did have significant intercept, $Z = 5.13, p < .0001$, and slope variance, $Z = 1.94, p = .0265$, but the covariance between slope and intercept was not significant. Reading comprehension for the group as a whole did not differ from the norm ($M = 99.25, SD = 9.7$) and change relative to the norm group was not significantly greater than zero ($M = .89, SD = 1.9$; see Figure 4). Reading comprehension levels were decelerating significantly, $t(69) = -2.75, p = .0077$.We would expect a 57% decline in slopes from 1 to 2 years postinjury.

Neither severity, age at injury, nor their interaction significantly predicted the rate of change (slope) or the deceleration (curvature). The interaction of severity and age at injury also failed to predict the level of reading comprehension at 1 year

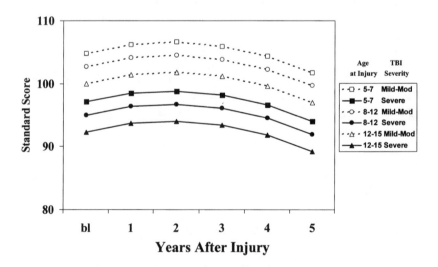

FIGURE 4   Expected values for growth curves for PIAT Reading Comprehension scores. The intercept parameter was significant, indicating that children with severe TBI scored lower than those with mild–moderate TBI. Neither the rate of change nor the deceleration of the growth curves over the follow-up was significant.

postinjury. The mild–moderate TBI group had significantly higher reading comprehension scores $(M = 105.0)$, $t(154) = 3.46$, $p = .0007$, than the severe TBI group $(M = 97.3)$, a difference of 0.88 SD. In addition, participants who were older at the time of injury tended to have lower reading comprehension scores, $t(154) = -1.69$, $p = .0928$. Severity and age at injury accounted for 17.2% of the variance in the intercepts and 12% of the total variance.

Analysis of Variance

Academic performance.   To evaluate academic functioning in the classroom, parent ratings of academic performance were obtained from the Child Behavior Checklist (1991) at 2 and 3 years after the injury (see Table 2). Analysis of variance revealed that children with severe TBI were rated as showing significantly poorer classroom performance than children with mild–moderate TBI that persisted 2, $F(1, 61) = 29.51$, $p < .0001$, and 3, $F(1, 37) = 8.00$, $p < .008$, years after injury.

Hierarchical Linear Regression Analyses

Hierarchical linear regression models were examined to determine the unique contribution of a set of neurological (duration of impaired consciousness), demographic (SES, gender), and neuropsychological variables to prediction of academic achievement scores and parent ratings of academic performance. In the first step, the durations of impaired consciousness, gender, and SES were entered and tested for significance. Gender did not contribute significantly to prediction of academic scores and was dropped from each model. In the second step, neuropsychological predictors were added to determine their unique contribution over and above variables on the first step. The unique R^2 for each variable and the total R^2 for each model are provided in Table 3.

TABLE 2
Academic Competence Scores From the Child Behavior Checklist at
2 and 3 Years After TBI

| | Severity of TBI | | | | | | |
| | Mild–Moderate | | Severe | | Statistics | | |
Follow-Up Interval	M	SD	M	SD	F	df	p
2 years t score	46.5	8.62	33.26	10.25	29.51	1, 61	.0001
3 years t score	46.7	8.19	36.39	10.39	8.00	1, 37	.008

Note.   TBI = traumatic brain injury.

TABLE 3
Hierarchical Regression Models of Achievement Variables

| | Unique R² | | | Model R² | |
| | Step 1 | | Step 2 | Total | |
Achievement Area	Coma	SES	Cognitive Predictors	R²	F(p)
WRAT arithmetic	.015	.002	NSR: .065*, DS: .014, VMI: .079*	.209	2.96*
WRAT spelling	.069*	.006	NSR: .000, VMI: .023, WF: .095***	.268	4.44***
WRAT reading	.125***	.056*	WF: .074**, RN: .086***	.418	11.87******
PIAT comprehension	.002	.001	RR: .012, VOC: .131**, DS: .012	.387	7.07******
School competence	.189******	.014	ABC: .075**, RC: .080***, AR: .031*	.629	15.23******

Note. SES = socioeconomic status; WRAT = Wide Range Achievement Test; NSR = nonverbal selective reminding; DS = Digit Span backwards; VMI = Beery Developmental Test of Visual-Motor Integration; WF = word fluency; RN = Rapid Automatized Naming Test; RR = WRAT Reading Recognition; VOC = Peabody Picture Vocabulary Test–Revised; ABC = Vineland Adaptive Behavior Composite score; RC = PIAT Reading Comprehension; AR = WRAT arithmetic.

*$p < .05$. **$p < .01$. ***$p < .005$. ****$p < .001$. *****$p < .0001$.

Academic Achievement Scores

Arithmetic.   Neither the duration of impaired consciousness nor SES predicted arithmetic scores. The consistent long-term retrieval score from the Nonverbal Selective Reminding Test and the Beery VMI score enhanced prediction and accounted for 6.5% and 7.9% of unique variance in the arithmetic scores, respectively. Contrary to expectation, the Digit Span backward variable did not explain additional variance in scores. The total model accounted for 20.9% of the variance in arithmetic scores.

Spelling.   The duration of impaired consciousness accounted for a modest proportion of variability in spelling scores. SES was not significantly related to the level of spelling performance. On step 2, neither the Nonverbal Selective Reminding score nor the Beery VMI score contributed significant unique variance. Word Fluency explained 9.5% of the variance in spelling scores, yielding a total model R^2 of .268.

Reading recognition.   In the first step, both coma and SES predicted the reading recognition score. For the second step, Word Fluency and Rapid Automatized Naming significantly enhanced prediction of word decoding. The variables included in step 2 accounted for an additional 19.4% of variance in reading recognition scores.

Reading comprehension.   Neither the duration of impaired consciousness nor SES predicted reading comprehension scores. As expected, the level of reading comprehension was significantly related to the level of vocabulary development. Neither Reading Recognition scores nor the backward Digit Span score enhanced prediction of the comprehension scores. Because the vocabulary and Reading Recognition variables were highly intercorrelated ($r = .66, p < .0001$), Reading Recognition did not contribute significant unique variance after vocabulary was entered into the model. The model R^2 was .387, indicating that a moderate amount of variation in comprehension scores was predicted by the cognitive variables.

Academic competence rating.   The duration of impaired consciousness accounted for 20% of variation in parent ratings of academic competence on the Child Behavior Checklist. Inclusion of SES did not improve prediction. Parent assessment of overall adaptive behaviors on the Vineland Adaptive Behavior Scales was significantly related to parent ratings of academic competence. Reading comprehension and arithmetic scores significantly enhanced prediction of parent ratings of academic performance. The total model R^2 was .629, indicating that the predictor variables accounted for a substantial proportion of variability in the ratings of academic competence. Similar to findings of Kinsella and colleagues (1997), long-term verbal memory scores did not predict academic competence as measured by parent ratings, $F(1, 58) = 0.06, p < .95$.

DISCUSSION

Academic achievement scores were examined in relation to severity of TBI, age at injury, and time since injury. Growth curve analysis identified robust relations with severity of injury, few relations with age at injury, and significant changes in the rate of growth of academic skills over time. Severity of TBI accounted for up to 13% of variability in the level of outcome and 16% of variability in the rate of change over time. Children and adolescents with severe brain injury received lower scores on tests of arithmetic, spelling, word decoding, and reading comprehension than those with mild to moderate brain injuries. The curve for spelling scores was relatively linear for the mild–moderate group as scores increased over the follow-up period. In contrast, spelling scores decelerated in the severe TBI group, suggesting less improvement over time.

The discrepancy between the academic achievement scores and parent ratings of academic performance was striking. Despite average achievement scores, the severe TBI group received low ratings of actual classroom performance at 2 and 3 years after the injury. Given adequate development of basic academic skills, it is likely that other cognitive and behavioral deficits contributed to poor classroom performance after severe TBI. Therefore, to assess specific areas of strength and weaknesses that impact the child's daily functioning, comprehensive individual assessments should include neuropsychological tests evaluating memory, attention, and processing speed, as well as measures of behavioral adjustment. To examine additional factors influencing performance, assessments should include measures of functional skills. Functional skills assessment is critically important to characterize the child's cognitive and behavioral strengths and weaknesses within the classroom as well as in less structured contexts such as free time or recess. Contextually valid assessment of performance should include conditions similar to those in the classroom setting, such as requirements for completion of tasks under time-limited conditions, the presence of realistic auditory and visual distractors, and expectations for self-directed initiation and completion of tasks (Ewing-Cobbs & Bloom, 2004; Ylvisaker et al., 2001). Better characterization of interrelations between academic, cognitive, and behavioral difficulties following TBI are needed to guide development of long-term intervention strategies.

The effect of age at injury varied across the different academic achievement tasks. The main effect for age was significant only for the arithmetic scores, which were lower in adolescents relative to younger children. However, age at injury also interacted with the rate of growth in skills for the arithmetic scores; scores were initially lower in adolescents and showed greater increases over time than scores from children. Importantly, the growth curves of the youngest children with both mild–moderate and severe TBI decelerated; scores decreased over the follow-up relative to the normative group and dropped from the average range at 1 to 2 years after TBI to the low average range by 5 years after TBI.

Hebb (1942) noted that organs in a rapid stage of development were more vulnerable to injury than developed organs. Our findings support the extension of Hebb's hypothesis to skill development as skills in a rapid stage of development appear to be especially vulnerable to the effects of injury (Ewing-Cobbs, Levin, Eisenberg, & Fletcher, 1987). We hypothesized that reading recognition scores would be most disrupted in younger children who are acquiring word-decoding skills and that later developing reading comprehension skills would be more disrupted in older children. Contrary to expectation, main effects of age and the age by severity interaction for reading recognition and reading comprehension scores were not significant. However, there was an interaction of age at injury with the slope or rate of growth of word-decoding skill; Reading Recognition scores increased more over time in older than in younger participants. By 5 years after the injury, the youngest children with severe TBI had the lowest scores of any age or severity groups. Although the mean scores remained average, the youngest children showed less adequate development of word-decoding skill over time. Reading comprehension scores tended to be lower in adolescents than children across the extended follow-up. Despite declines in word-decoding competence, younger children did not show concomitant decreases in comprehension scores. Our findings parallel those reported by Barnes et al. (1999), who found that word decoding was most disrupted in children who were less than 6.5 years at the time of injury, whereas reading comprehension was lowest in children less than 9 in comparison to older children and adolescents.

Longitudinal studies are essential to characterize the eventual impact of brain injury on later-developing academic, cognitive, and behavioral areas. The decelerating developmental trajectory of word-decoding and arithmetic skills in young children with TBI can only be identified through prospective, longitudinal follow-up evaluations that extend over many years. As indicated in this study, the consequences of brain injury may not be clearly manifest for several years following the injury. This is particularly true for young children, who must acquire many new skills despite injury to neural networks involved in attention, memory, and executive functions (Taylor & Alden, 1997).

When examined using hierarchical regression, the achievement scores had less consistent relations with the index of injury severity. The unique R^2 for the duration of impaired consciousness ranged from a low of .015 for the Arithmetic score to a high of .189 for the School Competence variable. The duration of impaired consciousness accounted for a significant amount of variability in the Spelling and Reading Recognition scores as well as the School Competence variable. In contrast, SES only accounted for 5.6% of the variance in word-decoding scores and did not account for significant variation in any other score. This finding is surprising because SES and estimates of family environment have been significantly related to academic variables in other studies of outcome from pediatric TBI. As noted by Yeates and colleagues (1997), direct measures of family functioning may be more strongly related to outcome after severe TBI than more indirect measures such as SES.

Concurrent cognitive–neuropsychological variables were predictive of academic achievement and the relations were generally consistent with models of reading decoding–spelling, reading comprehension, and arithmetic. Consistent with studies of math disability, Arithmetic scores were predicted by indexes of visual–spatial skill and visual memory; however, the working memory measure did not improve prediction. Word-decoding scores were strongly related to measures of phonological processing and automaticity in the retrieval of names for visual stimuli, which are the skills that are highly predictive of reading in both normal and reading-disabled groups. Similarly, spelling scores were predicted by the measure of phonological processing. Reading comprehension scores were predicted only by vocabulary knowledge. In contrast to Barnes et al. (1999), comprehension scores were not predicted by the level of word decoding. The predictors of reading comprehension scores were highly correlated; vocabulary knowledge likely subsumed shared variance.

It is interesting to note that, in previous longitudinal studies, growth curve modeling revealed that the adverse effects of severe pediatric TBI on Word Fluency (our measure of phonological processing in this study) persisted for at least 5 years without evidence of recovery to an age-appropriate level (Levin, Song, Ewing-Cobbs, Chapman, & Mendelsohn, 2001). In this study, Word Fluency accounted for significant unique variability in the word-decoding and spelling variables after controlling for measures of injury severity and preinjury SES. The estimate of working memory used in this study, the backward component of the Digit Span subtest, did not account for significant variation in arithmetic or reading comprehension scores. Inclusion of indexes of working memory in future studies that are derived from models of working memory may elucidate relations between working memory and complex academic skills following TBI (e.g., Hannon & Daneman, 2001; McLean & Hitch, 1992).

Interpretation of growth curves and longitudinal data is complicated by the difficulty equating assessments completed at different ages, which is partly related to the properties of the measures that are commonly used to assess academic achievement and which we have used here. First, many commonly used achievement tests have not been constructed using models of academic skill development and so they do not adequately measure the emergence of early academic skills in young children (see Ginsburg, Klein, & Starkey, 1998). The WRAT, for example, is known to have limited sensitivity in measuring arithmetic difficulties in children less than 8 years of age (Siegel & Ryan, 1989). Similarly, initial spelling items assess visual motor integration through letter formation whereas later items assess more phonologically based spelling skills. Second, time requirements on some tasks might have different implications for younger and older children. For example, on the arithmetic subtest, younger children are more likely to complete items within the time limit due to the fewer number of items within their capability, suggesting that for these children, the arithmetic subtest primarily measures arithmetic knowledge. In contrast, the performance of adolescents is dependent on both arithmetic knowledge and efficiency or speed with which arithmetic computations can be carried out. Given that significant reductions in motor speed and speed of information processing are characteristic deficits after severe TBI (Bawden, Knights, & Winogron, 1985; Thompson et al., 1994), the arithmetic subtest might be measuring somewhat different components of computational skills in adolescents than in younger children with TBI. Third, our measure of reading comprehension does not assess reading speed, which is known to be deficient in children with TBI and related to their reading comprehension (Barnes et al., 1999), nor does it distinguish between literal and inferential comprehension or measure the ability to integrate information across text (Barnes & Dennis, 2001).

Limitations of this study include the lack of longitudinal achievement scores from a comparison group of children without TBI. The lack of a comparison group may obscure developmental changes in the TBI groups, particularly in children with mild to moderate TBI. Replication of this study using a larger sample and a broader range of measures of academic skill development is needed. As this cohort of children was injured during the 1980s, replication with a contemporary cohort using current achievement measures would be helpful. The study would be enhanced by examination of the relation between specific neuroimaging findings and development of academic skills. Such an analysis would permit identification of specific risk factors, such as focal brain injury, that may impede the development of specific academic skills and interfere with the appropriate application of skills in everyday settings.

Future investigations should examine additional measures of academic skill development and should include functional assessment of academic skills. Emphasis should be placed on evaluation of cognitive subskills necessary for development of academic competence such as fluency and rate of word retrieval, phonological awareness, phonological and visual working memory, and sequencing skills. Additional variables of interest include self-management skills, metacognition, focused attention, and planning, as well as measures of discourse including summarization, inferencing, and gist recall. Moreover, relations between academic competence and measures of skills theoretically related to academic performance, such as deficits in executive functions, discourse, and self-management, should be assessed to characterize assets and liabilities that may influence academic skill development. Additional knowledge about the interrelations between academic skills and executive functions will also enhance the development of intervention strategies.

ACKNOWLEDGMENT

Preparation of this manuscript was supported in part by National Institutes of Health Grants RO1 HD–27597, RO1 NS–21889, and RO1 NS–29462.

REFERENCES

Achenbach, T. (1991). *Manual for the Child Behavior Checklist/4–18 and 1991 Profile.* Burlington, VT: University of Vermont College of Medicine.

Ackerman, P. T., & Dykman, R. A. (1995). Reading-disabled students with and without comorbid arithmetic disability. *Developmental Neuropsychology, 11,* 351–371.

Adams, M. J. (1990). *Beginning to read.* Cambridge, MA: MIT.

Barnes, M. A., & Dennis, M. (2001). Knowledge-based inferencing after childhood head injury. *Brain Injury, 76,* 253–265.

Barnes, M. A., Dennis, M., & Wilkinson, M. (1999). Reading after closed head injury in childhood: Effects on accuracy, fluency, and comprehension. *Developmental Neuropsychology, 15,* 1–24.

Bawden, H. N., Knights, R. M., & Winogron, H. W. (1985). Speeded performance following head injury in children. *Journal of Clinical and Experimental Neuropsychology, 7,* 39–54.

Beery, K. (1982). *Developmental test of visual–motor integration.* Cleveland, OH: Modern Curriculum.

Berger-Gross, P., & Shackelford, M. (1985). Closed head injury in children: Neuropsychological and scholastic outcomes. *Perceptual and Motor Skills, 61,* 254.

Bijur, P. E., Haslum, M., & Golding, J. (1990). Cognitive and behavioral sequelae of mild head injury in children. *Pediatrics, 86,* 337–344.

Bloom, D. R., Levin, H. S., Ewing-Cobbs, L., Saunders, A. E., Song, J., Fletcher, J. M., et al. (2001). Lifetime and novel psychiatric disorders after pediatric traumatic brain njury. *Journal of the American Academy of Child and Adolescent Psychiatry, 40,* 572–579.

Buschke, H. (1972). Components of verbal learning in children: Analysis by selective reminding. *Journal of Experimental Child Psychology, 18,* 488–496.

Chadwick, O., Rutter, M., Shaffer, D., & Shrout, P. E. (1981). A prospective study of children with head injuries: IV. Specific cognitive deficits. *Journal of Clinical Neuropsychology, 3,* 101–120.

Cohen, J. (1988). *Statistical power analysis for the behavioral sciences* (2nd ed.). Hillsdale, NJ: Lawrence Erlbaum Associates, Inc.

Denckla, M. B., & Rudel, G. R. (1976). Rapid automatized naming (R.A.N.): Dyslexia differentiated from other learning disabilities. *Neuropsychologia, 14,* 471–479.

Donders, J. (1994). Academic placement after traumatic brain injury. *Journal of School Psychology, 32,* 53–65.

Dunn, L., & Dunn, L. (1981). *Peabody Picture Vocabulary Test–Revised: Manual for forms L and M.* Circle Pines, MN: American Guidance Service.

Dunn, L., & Markwardt, F. (1970). *Peabody Individual Achievement Test.* Circle Pines, MN: American Guidance Service.

Ewing-Cobbs, L., & Bloom, D. R. (2004). Traumatic brain injury: Neuropsychological, psychiatric and educational issues. In R. T. Brown (Ed.), *Handbook of pediatric psychology in school settings* (pp. 313–331). Mahwah, NJ: Lawrence Erlbaum Associates, Inc.

Ewing-Cobbs, L., Fletcher, J. M., Levin, H. S., Iovino, I., & Miner, M. E. (1998). Academic achievement and academic placement following traumatic brain injury in children and adolescents: A two-year longitudinal study. *Journal of Clinical and Experimental Neuropsychology, 20,* 769–781.

Ewing-Cobbs, L., Levin, H. S., Eisenberg, H. M., & Fletcher, J. M. (1987). Language functions following closed-head injury in children and adolescents. *Journal of Clinical and Experimental Neuropsychology, 9,* 575–592.

Fay, G. C., Jaffe, K. M., Polissar, N. L., Liao, S., Martin, K. M., Shurtleff, H. A., et al. (1993). Mild pediatric traumatic brain injury: A cohort study. *Archives of Physical Medicine and Rehabilitation, 74,* 895–901.

Fay, G. C., Jaffe, K. M., Polissar, N. L., Liao, S., Rivara, J. B., & Martin, K. M. (1994). Outcome of pediatric traumatic brain injury at three years: A cohort study. *Archives of Physical Medicine and Rehabilitation, 75,* 733–741.

Fletcher, J. M. (1985). Memory for verbal and nonverbal stimuli in learning disability subgroups: Analysis by selective reminding. *Journal of Experimental Child Psychology, 40,* 244–259.

Fletcher, J. M., Ewing-Cobbs, L., Francis, D. J., & Levin, H. S. (1995). Variability in outcomes after traumatic brain injury in children: A developmental perspective. In S. H. Broman & M. E. Michel (Eds.), *Traumatic head injury in children* (pp. 3–21). New York: Oxford University Press.

Francis, D. J., Fletcher, J. M., Stuebing, K. K., Davidson, K., & Thompson, N. M. (1991). Analysis of change: Modeling individual growth. *Journal of Consulting and Clinical Psychology, 59,* 27–37.

Geary, D. C. (1993). Mathematical disabilities: Cognitive, neuropsychological and genetic components. *Psychological Bulletin, 114,* 345–362.

Gerring, J., Brady, K. D., Chen, A., Vasa, R., Gardos, M., Bandeen-Roche, K. J., et al. (1998). Premorbid prevalence of ADHD and development of secondary ADHD after closed head injury. *Journal of the American Academy of Child and Adolescent Psychiatry, 37,* 647–654.

Ginsburg, H. P., Klein, A., & Starkey, P. (1998). The development of children's mathematical thinking: Connecting research with practice. In I. E. Siegel & K. A. Renninger (Eds.), *Handbook of child psychology: Vol. 4, Child psychology in practice* (pp. 401–476). New York.

Gottardo, A., Stanovich, K. E., & Siegel, L. S. (1996). The relationships between phonological sensitivity, syntactic processing, and verbal working memory in the reading performance of third-grade children. *Journal of Experimental Child Psychology, 63,* 563–582.

Gough, P. B., Hoover, W. A., & Peterson, C. L. (1996). Some observations on a simple view of reading. In C. Cornoldi & J. Oakhill (Eds.), *Reading comprehension difficulties* (pp. 1–13). Mahwah, NJ: Lawrence Erlbaum Associates, Inc.

Hannon, B., & Daneman, M. (2001). A new tool for measuring and understanding individual differences in the component processes of reading comprehension. *Journal of Educational Psychology, 93,* 103–128.

Hebb, D. O. (1942). The effect of early and late brain injury upon test scores, and the nature of normal adult intelligence. *Proceedings of the American Philosophical Society, 85,* 275–292.

Hinshaw, S. P. (1992). Externalizing behavior problems and academic underachievement in childhood and adolescence: Causal relationships and underlying mechanisms. *Psychological Bulletin, 111,* 127–155.

Hollingshead, A. (1975). *Four factor index of social status.* Unpublished manuscript, Yale University.

Jaffe, K. M., Gayle, C. F., Polissar, N. L., Martin, K. M., Shurtleff, H. A., Rivara, J. B., et al. (1992). Severity of pediatric traumatic brain injury and early neurobehavioral outcome: A cohort study. *Archives of Physical Medicine and Rehabilitation, 73,* 540–547.

Jaffe, K. M., Gayle, C. F., Polissar, N. L., Martin, K. M., Shurtleff, H. A., Rivara, J. B., et al. (1993). Severity of pediatric traumatic brain injury and neurobehavioral recovery at one year: A cohort study. *Archives of Physical Medicine and Rehabilitation, 74,* 587–595.

Jastak, J. F., & Jastak, S. (1978). *The Wide Range Achievement Test manual of instructions.* Wilmington, DE: Jastak.

Kinsella, G. J., Prior, M., Sawyer, M., Murtagh, D., Einsenmajer, R., Anderson, V., et al. (1995). Neuropsychological deficit and academic performance in children and adolescents following traumatic brain injury. *Journal of Pediatric Psychology, 20,* 753–767.

Kinsella, G. J., Prior, M., Sawyer, M., Ong, B., Murtagh, D., Eisenmajer, R., et al. (1997). Predictors and indicators of academic outcome in children 2 years following traumatic brain injury. *Journal of the International Neuropsychological Society, 3,* 608–616.

Knights, R. M., Iran, L. P., Ventureyra, E. C., Bentirogrio, C., Stoddart, C., Winogron, H. W., et al. (1991). The effects of head injury in children on neuropsychological and behavioral functioning. *Brain Injury, 5,* 339–351.

Lennox, C., & Siegel, L. S. (1996). The development of phonological rules and visual strategies in average and poor spellers. *Journal of Experimental Child Psychology, 62,* 60–83.

Levin, H. S., & Benton, A. L. (1985). Developmental and acquired dyscalculia in children. In I. Flehmig (Ed.), *Second European Symposium on Developmental Neurology.* Stuttgart, Germany: Gustav Fischer Verlag.

Levin, H. S., & Ewing-Cobbs, L. (2001). Outcome for brain-injured children. In D. G. McLone, A. E. Marlin, R. M. Scott, P. Steinbok, D. H. Reigel, M. L. Walker, et al. (Eds.), *Pediatric neurosurgery* (4th ed., pp. 654–659). Philadelphia: W. B. Saunders.

Levin, H. S., Song, J., Ewing-Cobbs, L., Chapman, S. B., & Mendelsohn, D. (2001). Word fluency in relations to severity of closed head injury, associated frontal brain lesions, and age at injury in children. *Neuropsychologia, 39,* 122–131.

McLean, J. F., & Hitch, G. J. (1992). Working memory impairments in children with specific arithmetic learning difficulties. *Journal of Experimental Child Psychology, 74,* 240–260.

Michaud, L. J., Rivara, F. P., Jaffe, K. M., Fay, G. C., & Dailey, J. L. (1993). Traumatic brain injury as a risk factor for behavioral disorders in children. *Archives of Physical Medicine and Rehabilitation, 74,* 368–375.

Morris, R., Stuebing, K. K., Fletcher, J. M., Shaywitz, S. E., Lyon, G. R., Shankweiler, D., et al. (1998). Subtypes of reading disability: Variability around a phonological core. *Journal of Educational Psychology, 90,* 347–373.

Rivara, J. B., Jaffe, K. M., Polissar, N. L., Fay, G. C., Martin, K. M., Shurtleff, H. A., et al. (1994). Family functioning and children's academic performance and behavior problems in the year following traumatic brain injury. *Archives of Physical Medicine and Rehabilitation, 75,* 369–379.

Rivera-Batiz, F. L. (1992). Quantitative literacy and the likelihood of employment among young adults in the United States. *The Journal of Human Resources, 27,* 313–328.

Rourke, B. P. (1993). Arithmetic disabilities, specific and otherwise. *Journal of Learning Disabilities, 26,* 214–226.

Sattler, J. M. (1992). *Assessment of children.* San Diego, CA: San Diego State University.

Share, D. L., Moffit, T. E., & Silva, P. A. (1998). Factors associated with arithmetic-and-reading disability and specific arithmetic disability. *Journal of Learning Disabilities, 21,* 313–320.

Siegel, L. S., & Ryan, E. (1989). The development of working memory in normally achieving and subtypes of learning disabled children. *Child Development, 60,* 973–980.

Sparrow, S. S., Balla, D. A., & Cicchetti, D. V. (1984). *Vineland Adaptive Behavior Scales.* Circle Pines, MN: American Guidance Service.

Spreen, O. (1988). *Learning disabled children growing up: A follow up into adulthood.* New York: Oxford University Press.

Spreen, O., & Benton, A. L. (1969). *Neurosensory Center Comprehensive Examination for Aphasia: Manual of directions.* Victoria, British Columbia, Canada: Neuropsychology Laboratory, University of Victoria.

Stallings, G. A., Ewing-Cobbs, L., Francis, D. J., & Fletcher, J. M. (1995). Achievement test scores in head-injured children before and after injury. *Journal of International Neuropsychological Society, 1,* 156.

Taylor, H. G., & Alden, J. (1997). Age-related differences in outcomes following childhood brain insults: An introduction and overview. *Journal of the International Neuropsychological Society, 3,* 555–567.

Taylor, H. G., Yeates, K. O., Wade, S. L., Drotar, D., & Klein, S. (1999). Influences on first-year recovery from traumatic brain injury in children. *Neuropsychology, 13,* 76–89.

Taylor, H. G. Yeates, K. O. Wade, S. L., Drotar, D., Stancin, T., & Burant, C. (2001). Birdirectional child–family influences on outcomes of traumatic brain injury in children. *Journal of the International Neuropsychological Society, 7,* 755–767.

Taylor, H. G., Yeates, K. O., Wade, S. L., Drotar, D., Stancin, T., & Minich, N. (2002). A prospective study of short- and long-term outcomes after traumatic brain injury in children: Behavior and achievement. *Neuropsychology, 16,* 15–27.

Teasdale, G., & Jennett, B. (1974). Assessment of coma and impaired consciousness: A practical scale. *Lancet, 2,* 81–84.

Thompson, N. M., Francis, D. J., Stuebing, K. K., Fletcher, J. M., Ewing-Cobbs, L., Miner, M. E., et al. (1994). Motor, visual-spatial, and somatosensory skills after closed head injury in children and adolescents: A study of change. *Neuropsychology, 8,* 333–342.

van der Vlugt, H., & Satz, P. (1985). Subgroups and subtypes of learning-disabled and normal children: A cross-cultural replication. In B. P. Rourke (Ed.), *Neuropsychology of learning disabilities: Essentials of subtype analysis* (pp. 212–227). New York: Guilford.

Wagner, R. K., Torgesen, J. K., & Rashotte, C. A. (1994). Development of reading-related phonological processing abilities: New evidence of bidirectional causality from a latent variable longitudinal study. *Developmental Psychology, 30,* 73–87.

Wechsler, D. (1974). *Wechsler Intelligence Scale for Children: Revised.* New York: Psychological Corporation.

Wolf, M., & Bowers, P. G. (1999). The double deficit hypothesis for the developmental dyslexias. *Journal of Educational Psychology, 91,* 415–438.

Wrightson, P., McGinn, V., & Gronwall, D. (1995). Mild head injury in preschool children: Evidence that it can be associated with persisting cognitive defect. *Journal of Neurology, Neurosurgery, and Psychiatry, 59,* 375–380.

Yeates, K. O., Taylor, H. G., Drotar, D., Wade, S. L., Klein, S., Stancin, T., et al. (1997). Preinjury family environment as a determinant of recovery from traumatic brain injuries in school-age children. *Journal of the International Neuropsychological Society, 3,* 617–630.

Ylvisaker, M., Todis, B., Glang, A., Urbanczyk, M. S., Franklin, C., DePompei, R., et al. (2001). Educating students with TBI: Themes and recommendations. *Journal of Head Trauma Rehabilitation, 16,* 76–93.

DEVELOPMENTAL NEUROPSYCHOLOGY, 25(1&2), 135–158
Copyright © 2004, Lawrence Erlbaum Associates, Inc.

Ecological Assessment of Executive Function in Traumatic Brain Injury

Gerard A. Gioia
Pediatric Neuropsychology Program
Children's National Medical Center
Departments of Pediatrics and Psychiatry and Behavioral Sciences
George Washington University School of Medicine

Peter K. Isquith
Departments of Pediatrics and Psychiatry
Dartmouth Hitchcock Medical Center
Hanover, NH

Executive dysfunction is a common outcome in children who have sustained traumatic brain injury (TBI). Appropriate assessment of these complex interrelated regulatory functions is critical to plan for the necessary interventions yet present a challenge to our traditional methodologies. Ecological validity has become an increasingly important focus in neuropsychological assessment with particular relevance for the executive functions, which coordinate one's cognitive and behavioral capacities with real-world demand situations. The Behavior Rating Inventory of Executive Function (BRIEF) was developed to capture the real-world behavioral manifestations of executive dysfunction. Its development and various forms of validity, including ecological validity, are described. Application of the BRIEF's methodology to the assessment of executive dysfunction in TBI is provided. We advocate a multilevel approach to understanding executive function outcome in TBI, including traditional test-based measures of executive function, real-world behavioral manifestation of executive dysfunction, and the environmental system factors that impact the child. In this model, ecologically valid assessment of executive dysfunction provides an important bridge toward understanding the impact of component-level (i.e., test-based) deficits on the child's everyday adaptive functioning, which can assist the definition of targets for intervention.

Requests for reprints should be sent to Gerard A. Gioia, Pediatric Neuropsychology Program, Children's National Medical Center, Departments of Pediatrics and Psychiatry and Behavioral Sciences, George Washington University School of Medicine, 14801 Physicians Lane, Suite 173, Rockville, MD 20850. E-mail: ggioia@cnmc.org

The executive functions are a critically important area of neuropsychological function in the developing child. These neuropsychological mechanisms of regulatory control play fundamental roles in the child's cognitive, behavioral, and social–emotional development. The level of executive function, whether intact or impaired, has substantial implications for everyday social and academic function. Individuals with traumatic brain injury (TBI) have documented difficulties with executive function on tests of executive performance, such as inhibition, planning, behavioral regulation (Dennis, Guger, Roncadin, Barnes, & Schachar, 2001; Levin et al., 1996). But the challenge in assessing executive dysfunction is not only to find appropriate performance measures, as Lezak (1995) and others suggested, but also to evaluate the functional, real-world impact of executive dysfunction expressed in everyday activities. In this article, we address the assessment of the executive functions from a perspective that is different from the traditional performance-based test methodology. We approach this problem from an ecological perspective, using the everyday behavior of the child as reported by his or her parents and teachers.

Preparatory to exploring an ecological approach to the assessment of executive function in TBI, we will first review the neuropsychological deficits that result from TBI in children. We then turn our attention to the definition of the complex neuropsychological domain known as the executive functions. Next, we examine the challenges inherent in the assessment of executive functions. A discussion of the ecological validity of neuropsychological assessment, in general, and executive functions, in particular, ensues. We explore various traditional methods that have been used to assess the ability to manage and regulate behavior and cognition. The substance of the article is new work with our Behavior Rating Inventory of Executive Function (BRIEF) (Gioia, Isquith, Guy, & Kenworthy, 2000) as an ecologically valid model to assess children's executive functions. Finally, we discuss recent work that has applied the use of the BRIEF with children who have sustained TBI.

NEUROPSYCHOLOGICAL DEFICITS IN TBI

A variety of cognitive and behavioral deficits can result from traumatic injury to the developing brain, including deficits in attention, memory, processing speed, and executive functions (e.g., Anderson, Catroppa, Rosenfeld, Haritou & Morse, 2000; Asarnow, Satz, Light, & Neumann, 1991; Dennis, Barnes, Donnelly, Wilkinson, & Humphreys, 1996; Ewing-Cobbs et al., 1998; Fletcher, Ewing-Cobbs, Miner, Levin, & Eisenberg, 1990). Executive function deficits have been tied to a lack of integrity of the frontal lobes of the brain. Magnetic resonance imaging studies of the pathophysiology of TBI suggest particular vulnerability of the frontal (i.e., dorsolateral cortex, orbitofrontal cortex, and frontal white matter) and anterior temporal lobes (Levin et al., 1993). Some data have addressed the relation between frontal lobe damage and executive function subdomains. Children frequently exhibit neuropsychological difficulties associated with damage to the prefrontal regions with specific deficits in the executive functions such as planning, cognitive flexibility (Ylvisaker, Szekeres, & Hartwick, 1992), behavioral inhibition, and poor organization of learning, memory, and language formulation (Scheibel & Levin, 1997; Ylvisaker, 1998). Severity of TBI is related to specific deficits in executive functioning, such as planning, whereas injury to different regions of the frontal lobes results in different patterns of performance (Levin et al., 1994).

Related observations of real-world function in children with TBI suggest that executive function deficits may be related to functional competence at home and in the classroom, as well as to social cognitive and social affective functioning (Dennis et al., 2001). In real-world settings, children with TBI are at increased risk for experiencing significant difficulties with academic performance, emotional regulation, and social interaction (Eslinger 1998; Eslinger, Biddle, & Grattan, 1997; Eslinger & Grattan, 1991). Among children with TBI, the greatest impact of executive deficits may not be seen at the time of injury, but may emerge later with the dramatic increase in environmental, academic, behavioral, emotional, and social demands on the executive system during adolescence. Problems in social functioning for this group are often the most distinctive features (Ackerly, 1964; Dennis et al., 2001; Eslinger, 1998; Eslinger & Damasio, 1985; Marlowe, 1992). Executive function deficits can result in a demanding, self-centered personality, lack of social tact, impulsive speech and behaviors, disinhibition, apathy and indifference, or a lack of empathy (Eslinger, 1998).

The impact of executive dysfunction may be amplified, rather than attenuated, with increasing time since injury (Dennis, 2000). Prospective case studies (Ackerly, 1964; Grattan & Eslinger, 1991) show the onset of marked behavioral, social, and emotional problems in adolescents who sustained, and appeared to "recover" from, brain injury as children. To the extent that executive dysfunction is expressed both as poor test performance and as real-world dysfunction, it is important to have broad-based assessment tools that measure executive dysfunction in both contexts. As we will explore further, structured performance-based tests may not capture the full spectrum of real-world executive dysfunction, yet an understanding of such deficits and how they impact the child on a daily basis is necessary for developing successful interventions and accommodations. Appropriate intervention thus requires a full ecologically valid assessment of these complex, regulatory functions.

DEFINITION OF THE EXECUTIVE FUNCTIONS

Definitions and models of executive function are plentiful in the literature (e.g., Anderson, 1998; Barkley, 2000; Brown, 1999; Denckla, 1994; Dennis, 1991; Fuster, 1989; Goldman-Rakic, 1987; Levin et al., 1991; Stuss & Benson, 1986;

Welsh & Pennington, 1988), with varying degrees of overlap and consensus as to the overall nature of executive function and specific subdomains. We define the executive functions as a collection of related yet distinct abilities that provide for intentional, goal-directed, problem-solving action. Most would agree that the term is an umbrella construct defined as the control, supervisory, or self-regulatory functions that organize and direct all cognitive activity, emotional response, and overt behavior. Some authors argued, in fact, that it may not be possible to partition the central executive beyond the molar level (Burgess, 1997; Goldman-Rakic 1987), whereas others argued for varying degrees of fractionation (Burgess, Alderman, Evans, Emslie, & Wilson, 1998). Fuster (1985) discussed the critical subfunctions of the prefrontal cortex, that is, the executive functions, necessary for performing long-term goal-directed tasks via the mediation of contingencies across time. Such executive functions are highlighted by delayed tasks, which require the ability to hold information actively in mind in the service of a future goal. Three key components of this system are described, including the following:

- The temporally retrospective function of working memory, the ability to hold old information in mind while actively processing new information.
- The temporally prospective function of anticipatory set.
- Control of interference, which includes the ability to inhibit competing information and action.

Stuss and Benson (1986) described a set of related capacities for intentional problem solving including anticipation, goal selection, planning, monitoring, and use of feedback. Their hierarchical model highlights important aspects of the executive functions that relate to the highest levels of cognition, including anticipation, judgment, self-awareness, and decision making. Welsh and Pennington (1988) provided an early examination of the developmental aspects of the executive functions in children. They characterized the development of the executive functions in terms of "the ability to maintain an appropriate problem-solving set for attainment of a future goal" (p. 201). Finally, Denckla (1994) defined the critical features of the executive functions for active problem solving as follows: providing for delayed responding, future-oriented, strategic action selection, intentionality, anticipatory set, freedom from interference, and the ability to sequence behavioral outputs. Despite the use of different terminology and different emphases in the definitions of these various authors, the common feature amont them is the executive system as a set of supervisory functions enabling regulatory control over thought and actions.

Most authors view the executive functions as a set of interrelated capacities rather than as a unitary function. In reviewing the list of domains discussed by others, we have arrived at a basic set of behaviorally referenced areas. Specific subdomains that make up this collection of regulatory or management functions include the abilities to initiate behavior, inhibit competing actions or stimuli, select relevant task goals, plan and organize a means to solve complex problems, shift problem-solving strategies flexibly when necessary, and monitor and evaluate one's own behavior. The working memory capacity to hold information actively "online" in the service of problem solving is also described within this domain of functioning (Pennington, Bennetto, McAleer, & Roberts, 1996). Finally, we believe the executive functions are not exclusive to cognition; emotional control is also reciprocally related to effective problem-solving activity. That is, goal-oriented problem solving requires not only cognitive control but also the appropriate regulation of one's affective state.

Although we define the executive functions as specific self-regulatory behaviors, it is crucial to understand how these functions operate. In this conceptualization, the executive functions serve as an integrated directive system exerting regulatory control over the basic, domain-specific neuropsychological functions (e.g., language, visuospatial functions, memory, emotional experience, motor skills) in the service of a reaching an intended goal. The executive system makes active, intentional decisions regarding the final behavioral output and recruits the necessary components to reach the goal. As such, the executive functions are defined as the control or self-regulatory functions that organize and direct all cognitive activity, emotional response, and overt behavior. One must approach the assessment process differently depending on whether problem-solving deficits are the result of deficient basic functions (e.g., language) versus a faulty executive control mechanism. The two must work together to produce a coherent, goal-directed product but each has a fundamentally different role toward this end. The unique directive, regulatory nature of the executive functions calls for distinctive methods of assessment.

ASSESSMENT OF EXECUTIVE FUNCTION

Though the executive functions may be defined in a relatively straightforward manner, their precise assessment can be very challenging. A clear understanding of the differences between assessment of the "basic" domain-specific content areas of function (e.g., memory, language, visuospatial, social–emotional) and the domain general or "control" aspects of cognition and behavior is essential. What may appear as a problem with the expression of language may be due less (or not at all) to the basic aspects of linguistic functioning (e.g., phonology, syntax, semantics) than to poor "meta-linguistic" functions (e.g., formulating and maintaining an organized, planful approach to the topic of conversation). There is no test or battery that singularly assesses executive function. By necessity, there is always a "domain-specific" content area regulated by the executive control process. Teasing apart executive functions from domain-specific functions is part of the challenge of the neuropsychological assessment. Efforts to operationalize assessment models of executive function have largely focused on laboratory or clinical performance tests (Kelly, 2000; Welsh & Pennington, 1988; Welsh, Pennington, & Grossier, 1991), with their inherent construct and measurement problems (Pennington et al., 1996; Rabbit, 1997). For example, Burgess (1997) suggested that most neuropsychological tests alone are inadequate in assessing the executive functions because they attempt to separate integrated functions into component parts. Many consider the Wisconsin Card Sorting Task (Heaton, Chelune, Talley, Kay, & Curtiss, 1993) the prototypical test of executive function, despite the inherently limited focus and scope of any single performance measure. Yet, in their comprehensive review of executive function and ADHD studies, Pennington and Ozonoff (1996) cited only a few performance tests that are consistently impaired across studies and note that the Wisconsin Card Sorting Test is not among them. Furthermore, current performance-based tests tap individual components of executive function over a short time frame and not the integrated, multidimensional, relativistic, priority-based decision-making that is often demanded in real-world situations (Goldberg & Podell, 2000; Shallice & Burgess, 1991). As a result, narrow-band, component tests may not be sufficient in capturing more complex, day-to-day, executive problem solving. The need exists for ecologically valid tasks that assess the broader, molar aspects of complex, everyday, problem-solving demands.

ECOLOGICAL VALIDITY IN NEUROPSYCHOLOGICAL ASSESSMENT

The shift over time in neuropsychological assessment from identifying brain injury and lesion location to describing functional strengths and weaknesses (Lezak, 1995) and to predicting everyday functioning and needs for intervention and support in the natural environment (Hart & Hayden, 1986; Long, 1996) has necessitated a parallel shift from "traditional" validity considerations (Franzen & Wilhelm, 1996) to ecological validity considerations. Ecological validity in the psychological literature refers in general to the ability to generalize results of controlled experiments to naturally occurring events in the real world (Brunswick, 1955). Regarding neuropsychological assessment, ecological validity may be more narrowly defined as the "functional and predictive relation between the patient's behavior on a set of neuropsychological tests and the patient's behavior in a variety of real-world settings" (Sbordone, 1996, p. 16). Thus, an ecologically valid assessment tool is one that has characteristics similar to a naturally occurring behavior and has value in predicting everyday function (Franzen & Wilhelm, 1996).

When neuropsychological tests are developed and applied to identify or quantify deficits, traditional validity (e.g., construct validity) is paramount and ecological validity may be of little concern. In practice, however, neuropsychologists are increasingly asked to not only identify functional strengths and weaknesses but to translate such findings into implications and predictions for the individual in his or her everyday milieu. Particularly complex are the demands placed on pediatric neuropsychologists, who are asked what the child's strengths and weaknesses are, along with questions about academic placement, needed interventions and accommodations, appropriate IEP goals, implications for school and community functioning, and what future behavioral and emotional developments might be expected in the course of that child's development (Silver, 2000). In this scenario, ecological validity becomes paramount.

Implicit in definitions of ecological validity as the concept is applied to neuropsychological assessment are two requirements: first, that the demands of a test and the testing conditions resemble demands in the everyday world of the child; second, that performance on a test predicts some aspect of the child's functioning on a day-to-day basis. The first requirement, that of *verisimilitude*, overlaps with face validity and describes the "topographical similarity" or theoretical relation between the method of data collection and skills or behaviors required in the natural environment of the child (Franzen & Wilhelm, 1996). For example, to what degree does a test that requires scanning a page and crossing out symbols or pictures resemble a child's activity in school or at home? Some traditional tests have arguably greater verisimilitude in this regard, such as list learning, prose memory, or naming tasks, whereas the relation between copying a complex figure or sorting cards by category and everyday activities is less transparent.

Considerations of verisimilitude include not only the demands of a given test itself but also the conditions in which the test is administered. That is, in evaluating the degree of verisimilitude for a given test, both the required skills and the testing environment and methods need to be considered. For example, though listening to and repeating a list of objects or words bears theoretical resemblance to learning that might be required in school, the controlled rate of presentation, nondistracting assessment setting and environmental structure, guided practice over several trials, and cues to organize the information may not approximate real-world demands. Although such administrative controls and structure are necessary in the assessment setting to ensure reliability and internal validity, they may compromise ecological validity. Indeed, the more likely environment where listening and remembering is required is one in which there are distractions, the presentation rate is varied, there is limited opportunity for rehearsal, and there may be additional demands such as taking notes. Tests administered within the confines and controls of the laboratory setting may thus underestimate the implications of a child's difficulties or deficits in the classroom. On the other hand, such tests may overestimate functional difficulties, as the child may apply compensatory strategies in their everyday world or exhibit behavior patterns that increase functionality (Ylvisaker & Gioia, 1998).

The second requirement of ecological validity in neuropsychological assessment is *veridicality*, or the degree to which test performance predicts some aspect of the child's everyday functioning. This aspect is both theoretical and empirical: Theoretically, is there reason to believe the test might predict real-world behavior; and empirically, does test performance correlate with some measure of real-world functioning (Franzen & Wilhelm, 1996; Rabin, 2001)? Though this has been the focus of increasing attention, very little is known about prediction of everyday behavior from neuropsychological tests. Methodologically, such an analysis is complicated by the difficulties inherent in capturing an individual's functioning in a reliable and valid numerical fashion. In the adult literature, several studies have focused on the correlation of neuropsychological test data with patients' vocational status (e.g., Bayless, Varney, & Roberts, 1989), or, more commonly, with rating scales that assess aspects of daily functioning (Dunn, Searight, Grisso, Margolis, & Gibbons, 1990) or vocational functioning (e.g., Lysaker, Bell, & Beam-Goulet, 1995).

Assessment of veridicality in pediatric neuropsychology is further complicated by confounds unique to children. Silver (2000) cogently articulated four primary challenges to assessing the ecological validity of child-focused assessment instruments: methodology of neuropsychological assessment, methodology of assessing everyday functioning, developmental factors, and intervening variables. Whereas the first two issues are inherently problematic in both adult and child assessment, the latter two are unique to, or more complex in, pediatric populations. Developmental considerations introduce variability, dampening the predictive power of neuropsychological tests (Silver, 2000). At one level, we are simply unable to perform detailed assessment of the full spectrum of typical neuropsychological domains in very young children, and even if we could, it is not clear that tests developed for adults or older children tap similar functions in younger children. Because executive functions are tied to emergent development, the status of executive function in children with perturbations of development need to be tied to the developmental stage of the child at perturbation or brain insult. At another level, children are still developing and functions are emerging into early adulthood. Thus, it may not be possible to detect or evaluate functional difficulties or to assess their impact on everyday functioning until the child matures. In the case of children with TBI or other acquired insult, deficits may not become apparent until the environment places demands on a particular function.

Finally, intervening variables may influence the ability to assess ecological validity to a greater extent with children. The child's environment is such a mediator: Family environment is affected by a child's functional difficulties, and the family environment in turn affects the child (Taylor et al., 1999). Further, a child with neuropsychological deficits may receive additional supports, either through developmental or rehabilitation services or through the school. Indeed, Silver (2000) noted a paradox in ecological validity determination with child instruments: Once weaknesses are identified via neuropsychological assessment, recommendations are generally proffered for interventions with a goal of ameliorating the functional deficits to enhance everyday functioning, thus modifying the statistical relation between the original tests and future measures of everyday functioning.

ECOLOGICAL VALIDITY AND ASSESSMENT OF EXECUTIVE FUNCTION

The methodology of neuropsychological assessment places particular constraints on assessment of executive function. The structured and interactive nature of the typical assessment situation may relieve the demands on the executive functions, and thereby reduce the opportunity to observe critical behaviors associated with the executive functions (Bernstein & Waber, 1990). That is, in many testing situations, the examiner provides the structure, organization, guidance, plan, cueing, and monitoring necessary for optimal performance by the child, thereby serving as that child's external executive control (Kaplan, 1988; Stuss & Benson, 1986). A child with significant executive dysfunction can perform appropriately on well-structured tasks of knowledge in which the examiner is allowed to cue and probe for more information, thus relieving the child of the need to be strategic and goal directed, or to exercise their executive functions more generally.

Recognizing the different stimulus conditions that are provided within the comfort of the controlled setting of testing (which may be necessary to identify the child's knowledge and abilities) versus those existing within the child's everyday world is critically important. Frequently, the more novel or complex the task, the greater the demand for the executive functions. The more familiar, automatic, and simple the task, the less the child needs to recruit his or her executive functions. What may be a complex, novel task for one child may be a relatively familiar and automatic task for another, requiring that such children recruit vastly different degrees of executive control functions toward solving that particular problem. The ultimate application of assessment data to formulating credible practical recommendations and intervention strategies demands a clear understanding of this issue. Assessing the child's behavior and responses under greater and lesser degrees of examiner-determined control and structure can help clarify the child's executive control competence.

A paradox in the assessment of the executive functions is that some individuals with significant deficits in specific executive function subdomains may, in fact, perform appropriately on many purported "tests of executive function," yet have significant problems making simple real-life decisions (Stuss & Buckle, 1992). All tests are multifactorial, requiring for any particular individual greater or lesser degrees of domain-specific content knowledge and experience (the novelty-familiarity issue), and thereby demanding varying degrees of organization, planning, inhibitory control, and flexibility. For example, a child may be able to perform appropriately on the Wisconsin Card Sorting Test (Heaton et al., 1993), which requires flexibility in problem solving, yet fail miserably in strategically modifying his or her approach to completing a set of math problems in the classroom. Goldberg and Podell (2000) argued that many existing neuropsychological tests assess more narrow veridical than real-world adaptive decision-making; as a result, one may not be collecting the relevant data to document the full essence of strengths and weaknesses in the array of executive functions.

The past decade has seen attention to ecological validity in assessment of executive function and the development of new assessment devices with verisimilitude in mind (Lezak, 1982; Roberts, Franzen, Furuseth, & Fuller, 1995; Shallice & Burgess, 1991; Wilson, Evans, Emslie, Alderman, & Burgess, 1998). Whereas increased attention to verisimilitude in test development and to demonstrating the veridicality of these newer measures and existing tests of executive function is reported in the adult assessment-focused literature (e.g., Bayless, Varney, & Roberts, 1989; Burgess, Alderman, Wilson, Evans, & Emslie, 1996; Kibby, Schmitter-Edgecombe, & Long, 1998; Lysaker, Bell, & Beam-Goulet, 1995), less attention has been paid to similar issues in the pediatric assessment literature. In her comprehensive review of ecological validity in neuropsychological assessment of children with TBI, Silver (2000) noted the multiple challenges to establishing ecological validity in this context. The majority of studies reviewed predict neuropsychological test variables from injury characteristics (e.g., Glasgow Coma Scale), rather than postinjury functioning from neuropsychological test variables, as though performance on neuropsychological tests is an outcome in and of itself. Several more recent studies, however, examine the relations between test performance and functioning in the everyday context via rating scales or structured interviews such as the Vineland Adaptive Behavior Scales (Sparrow, Balla, & Cicchetti, 1984) or via academic achievement testing as a proxy for school functioning (Hartlage & Templer, 1996). Regarding measures of executive function, there is precedent for the use of rating scales designed to tap executive functions in the everyday environment and promise in their use for demonstrating veridicality (Goulden, Silver, Harward, & Levin, 1997; Isquith & Gioia, 1999; Molho & Silver, 1997). Silver concluded that, despite the current limitations to ecological validity, neuropsychological tests are necessary to inform the clinician as to strengths and weaknesses under the best of circumstances to "illuminate the individual ability profile upon which interventions should be based" (p. 986).

In sum, as neuropsychologists are increasingly asked to make predictions about a child's functioning in the everyday environment and to recommend interventions and accommodations, demonstrating, or increasing, the ecological validity of our testing repertoire becomes essential. One consideration involves developing new measures from an ecological perspective, with particular attention to verisimilitude or similarity to real-world tasks. Given the challenges inherent in such novel test development, an alternative or parallel course is to examine the ability of our existing tool kit to predict children's functioning in the everyday environment, or it's veridicality. This is not without impediments, including the very methodology of neuropsychological tests and testing, the methodology of functional assessment, the developmental course of the subjects, and the likelihood of intervening variables. Despite the challenges, there are potential, if not promising, avenues of research and development in the service of ecologically valid assessment of executive function, and more broadly, of pediatric neuropsychological assessment in general. One avenue is to develop future tests with an emphasis on verisimilitude, such as the Test of Everyday Attention for Children (Manly, Robertson, Anderson, & Nimmo-Smith, 1999). Another avenue is to develop better methods to reliably capture aspects of children's everyday functioning in specific domains, such as the executive functions, that enable assessment of veridicality. A third avenue that may balance the conflicting validity demands of performance tests with the ecological validity demands of assessment applications is to develop both avenues concomitantly: traditional tests of discrete neuropsychological functions administered in well-controlled settings to preserve construct validity and identify a child's profile along with reliable measures of these functions through ratings of everyday behaviors in the natural environment to enable greater confidence in predictions from neuropsychological assessment.

BRIEF

The BRIEF was developed with ecological validity in mind. The impetus for the BRIEF came from our own clinical need to more efficiently and systematically capture information about manifestations of executive function difficulties in children's everyday behaviors at home, in school, and in their communities. Parents and teachers possess a wealth of information about children's behavior in these settings that is directly relevant to an understanding of executive function. Historically, we gathered this information via lengthy interviews with parents, and often could not elicit similar input from teachers due to time constraints. A well-established tradition exists, however, in utilizing structured behavior rating systems in the assessment of psychological and neuropsychological functions (Achenbach, 1991; Conners, 1989; Reynolds & Kamphaus, 1994). Given the difficulties and complexities involved in performance assessment of executive function and a need for greater ecological validity in evaluating executive function, we developed BRIEF to assess the behavioral manifestations of executive functions in children aged 5 to 18 years (Gioia et al., 2000). The BRIEF was designed as a means of culling and standardizing the rich information provided by parents and teachers in a more reliable and efficient manner with known psychometric properties. Such an ecologically valid system of assessing the everyday self-regulatory behaviors of children serves as an integral component in the clinical evaluation of executive dysfunction.

The BRIEF assesses eight interrelated subdomains of executive function: Inhibit, Shift (Flexibility), Emotional Control, Initiate, Working Memory, Plan–Organize, Organization of Materials, and Monitor. These descriptors were selected from domains commonly discussed in the literature (e.g., Denckla, 1989; Stuss & Benson, 1986; Welsh, Pennington, & Grossier, 1991; Ylvisaker, Szekeres, & Hartwick, 1992) and from discussions with colleagues. More general domains of executive function (e.g., self-regulation, anticipation) for which specific behaviors could not be generated were not included. Other possible domains (e.g., goal setting, strategic problem solving) were incorporated within the eight existing domains (e.g., planning, shift). The eight domains and examples of their everyday behavioral manifestation are described as follows:

1. *Inhibit* is the ability to resist or delay an impulse, to appropriately stop one's own activity at the proper time, or both. The ability to inhibit is readily observed in daily activities such as acting without thinking, being easily distracted, and being unable to sit still.

2. *Shift* captures the ability to alter problem-solving strategy during complex tasks, the ability to think flexibly, and the ability to switch or alternate attention. In their day-to-day lives, children may exhibit problems with transitioning from one situation, activity, or aspect of a problem to another as the situation demands. Caregivers often describe these children as "getting stuck" on a topic, or as being highly perseverative.

3. *Emotional control* is the manifestation of executive function within the emotional realm. It is closely associated with the ability to inhibit and modulate responses. Emotional control is a characteristic that is not easily assessed in the laboratory, but can be readily observed at home and school. An inability to modulate emotional responses may manifest as overblown emotional reactions to seemingly minor events or as a general affective reactivity.

4. *Initiate* is described as the ability to begin a task or activity, or the process of generating ideas or problem-solving strategies. Caregivers often report that children with initiation difficulties have trouble getting started on homework or chores and that they require prompts or cues to begin. Problems with initiation are not the result of noncompliance or disinterest in the task: The child typically has an interest in the task or activity and wants to succeed but cannot get started.

5. *Working memory* is the process of holding information in mind for the purpose of completing a related task. Working memory is essential to follow complex instructions, complete mental arithmetic, or perform tasks with more than one step. A common observation is that a child with working memory difficulties has trouble remembering things for even a few minutes, or when sent to get something, forgets what she or he was supposed to get.

6. The ability to *plan* involves anticipating future events, setting goals, and developing appropriate steps ahead of time to carry out an associated task or action. Planning involves imagining or developing a goal or end state, and then strategically determining the most effective method or steps to attain that goal. This often involves the sequencing and stringing together of steps to most efficiently move toward an end state. Parents and teachers may complain about the child's lack of planning ability, tendency to start assignments at the last minute, or not thinking ahead about possible problems.

7. The ability to *organize* complex information becomes increasingly important as demands for independent functioning increase (Bernstein, the natural history of LD). Organization involves establishing and maintaining order within an activity or carrying out a task in a systematic manner. Caregivers may report observing a scattered approach to solving problems, that the child is easily overwhelmed by large tasks or assignments, or has difficulties organizing personal belongings.

8. The ability to *self-monitor* includes checking on one's own actions during or shortly after finishing a task to assure appropriate attainment of a goal. Children who do not self-monitor often rush through assignments without checking their work for mistakes. Additionally, such children may be unaware of how their actions affect others in a social context.

Specific items for the BRIEF scales were generated primarily from behavioral descriptions of executive difficulties during clinical interviews with parents and teachers, ensuring good face and content validity. Item-category membership was determined by the sorting decisions of 12 clinical neuropsychologists, as well as statistical analyses (item–total correlation analyses, principal factor analyses, and interrater agreement). Table 1 presents sample items within each subdomain along with item–total correlations, percentage of agreement amongst expert ratings as to item–scale fit, and Cronbach's (1951) alpha as an indicator of internal consistency for the parent and teacher forms of the BRIEF.

The resulting instrument demonstrates appropriate psychometric integrity. Internal consistency is high, with values ranging from .80 to .98. Test–retest reliability is adequate, with average correlations of .81 for parent clinical scales (.84–.88 for the index scores) in the normative sample over a two week period. Similarly, average teacher test–retest correlations for the clinical scales were .87 (.90–.92 for the index scores) over a 3.5-week period. Correlations between parent and teacher informants are moderate, with an overall mean of .32 for the normative sample, which is similar to the literature on consistency among parent–teacher informants (Achenbach, McConaughty, & Howell, 1987).

The construct validity of the BRIEF was examined using common factor analysis while exploring uni- versus multidimensional solutions. Parent ratings of 852 clinically referred and 1,419 children in the normative sample, and teacher ratings

TABLE 1

BRIEF Sample Scale Items, Item–Total Correlations, and Interrater Agreement for Parent and Teacher Forms

Scale	Sample Item Content	Parent Form Item–Total Correlations	Teacher Form Item–Total Correlations	Expert Ratings (%)
Inhibit	Interrupts others	.63	.82	100
	Gets out of seat at the wrong times	.65	.79	100
	Gets out of control more than friends	.70	.82	77
Shift	Resists accepting a different way to solve a problem with schoolwork, friends, chores, and so on	.52	.63	100
	Becomes upset with new situations	.62	.71	100
	Acts upset by a change in plans	.59	.72	100
Emotional control	Overreacts to small problems	.58	.73	100
	Has explosive, angry outbursts	.59	.75	100
	Mood changes frequently	.62	.79	100
Initiate	Is not a self-starter	.51	.73	100
	Needs to be told to begin a task even when willing	.48	.68	100
	Has trouble getting started on homework or chores	.54	.69	100
Working memory	When given three things to do, remembers only the first or last	.60	.72	88
	Has trouble concentrating on chores, schoolwork	.68	.77	88
	Needs help from adult to stay on task	.67	.78	100
Plan–organize	Does not bring home homework, assignment sheets, materials, and so on	.55	.67	100
	Has good ideas but cannot get them on paper	.57	.72	75
	Gets caught up in details and misses the big picture	.54	.58	100
Organization of materials	Cannot find things in room or school desk	.60	.82	100
	Leaves a trail of belongings wherever they go	.71	.77	100
	Leaves messes that others have to clean up	.69	.78	100
Monitor	Does not check work for mistakes	.49	.60	100
	Makes careless errors	.58	.61	100
	Is unaware of how his or her behavior affects or bothers others	.56	.57	100

Note. BRIEF = Behavior Rating Inventory of Executive Function.

of 475 clinically referred and 720 students in the normative sample were examined. The eight scales were submitted to a principal factor analysis with oblique rotation. Examination of one-, two-, three-, and four-factor solutions yielded a similar factor structure for the parent and teacher clinical and normative groups. The two-factor solution was the most theoretically and statistically sound. Across parent and teacher groups, Factor 1, a metacognitive problem-solving factor, was defined by the subdomains Initiate, Working Memory, Plan–Organize, Organization of Materials, and Monitor. Factor 2, a behavior regulation factor, was defined by Inhibit, Shift, and Emotional Control. Correlations between the two factors ranged from .56 to .71. The overall stability of the two-factor solutions across clinical and normative samples for the parent and teacher scales provided strong support for the underlying factor structure of the BRIEF. This analysis also provided support for a limited multidimensional model of executive function.

To establish a measure of convergent and discriminant validity, the BRIEF was examined in relation to general measures of behavior in children (Child Behavior Checklist [CBCL]–Teacher Report Form [TRF], Achenbach, 1991; Behavior Assessment System for Children [BASC]; Reynolds & Kamphaus, 1992). Principal factor analyses (PFA) of the BRIEF and general behavioral measures resulted in similar four-factor structures, with most of the BRIEF scales separating from the TRF–CBCL and BASC scales (Gioia, Isquith, & Guy, 1998). The BRIEF structure was again defined by a "metacognitive problem-solving" factor (BRIEF Initiate, Working Memory, Plan–Organize, Organization of Materials, Monitor scales (with Attention scale of CBCL–TRF and BASC), a "behavior regulation" factor (BRIEF Inhibit, Shift, Emotional Control along with BASC Aggression scale), a CBCL–TRF or BASC externalizing factor, and a CBCL–TRF or BASC "internalizing" factor.

Overall, the BRIEF has strong psychometric integrity. The instrument as a whole and the individual scales are face valid with good content validity, are internally consistent, and have appropriate reliability properties. Factor analyses provide support for a consistent two-factor structure of the BRIEF, for convergent validity, and for discriminant validity.

In examining the ecological validity of the BRIEF, recall that there are two considerations, verisimilitude and veridicality. To achieve verisimilitude, the demands of a test are to be similar to demands in the everyday world of the child; to achieve veridicality, the test performance must predict some aspect of the child's daily functioning. Regarding verisimilitude, the BRIEF was explicitly designed to capture everyday executive behaviors while balancing the demands for reliability and construct validity. Examples of items within the BRIEF clinical scales that attempt to capture the everyday manifestations of executive dysfunction include "Tries the same approach to a problem over and over even when it does not work" tapping problem-solving inflexibility or "When sent to get something, forgets what he or she is supposed to get" tapping working memory. Such items were selected to be a direct reflection of real-world difficulties encountered by dysexecutive children and thus address verisimilitude.

The BRIEF also shows promise for veridicality, that is, predicting behavior in the natural environment. The correlational analyses with the BRIEF scales and broad behavioral measures suggest strong, logical relations (e.g., the BRIEF Inhibit scale with the Aggressive Behavior scale on the CBCL and the Aggression scale on the BASC). There is some suggestion that BRIEF scores correlate with scholastic achievement (Mahone, Koth, Cutting, Singer, & Denckla, 2001), an indication of "real-world" functioning (Hartlage & Templer, 1996). Preliminary work by our group has also found significant and selective correlations between the BRIEF and children's everyday adaptive behavior functioning (Janusz, Ahluvalia, & Gioia, 2001). Finally, given that executive functions are the underlying neuropsychological constructs reflected in the diagnostic symptoms of ADHD (Barkley, 1997, 2000; Brown, 1999; Denckla, 1996; Isquith & Gioia 1999; Pennington & Ozonoff, 1996; Welsh & Pennington, 1988), the BRIEF should predicting ADHD subtype diagnosis. Indeed, two BRIEF scales that are theoretically related to ADHD symptoms—Working Memory and Inhibit—are strongly predictive of ADHD subtypes (Gioia & Isquith, in press; Isquith & Gioia, 2000).

ECOLOGICAL ASSESSMENT OF EXECUTIVE FUNCTION IN TBI

As previously noted, various types of executive dysfunction characterize the functional deficits seen in children with TBI (Ylvisaker, 1998). Problem-solving rigidity (Ylvisaker, Szekeres, & Hartwick, 1992), disinhibition, and planning deficits (Levin et al., 1994; Scheibel & Levin, 1997) have all been described. Most of the TBI literature has used performance-based tests in their identification of executive dysfunction. Few have examined the short-term recovery and long-term outcome from a broader ecologically relevant perspective (Silver, 2000). Notable exceptions exist, however. Taylor and Yeates have conducted a program of research (e.g., Taylor et al., 2001; Taylor et al., 1999; Yeates et al., 1997; Wade et al., 2001) in which family context variables are integrally examined regarding their relation to neuropsychological outcome. They report the influence of the preinjury family as a moderator variable on the outcome of TBI. The family environment and burden are discussed as critical factors to consider in understanding neuropsychological outcome with significant implications for interventions. Ylvisaker and Feeney (1998) have also championed a contextualized approach to the everyday manifestations of TBI, with a particular focus on the executive functions. In this model, the important caretakers (parents, teachers) take an active role in the assessment of the child's functional strengths and weaknesses and also play a critical role in the intervention programming. Recently, Dennis et al. (2001) examined parent ratings of attentional–inhibitory control and social–behavioral regulation in children with TBI in addition to neuropsychological performance testing. They report selective relations between testing and everyday behavior ratings.

The structure of the BRIEF has significant promise in the assessment of ecologically relevant aspects of executive dysfunction in TBI. The three subdomains of the *Behavioral Regulation* factor—Inhibit, Shift, and Emotional Control—are commonly reported problems following injury to the prefrontal regions of the brain. In addition, difficulties in executive function tapped by the five subdomains of the *Metacognition* factor—Initiate, Working Memory, Plan–Organize, Organization of Materials, and Monitor—can also result from TBI. One such study of executive functioning using the BRIEF in children who have sustained TBI was conducted by Armstrong, Mangeot, Colvin, Yeates, and Taylor (2001). The authors report on the long-term prevalence and correlates of executive dysfunction following childhood traumatic brain injuries. The children in their sample were approximately 5 years postinjury, including severe and moderate TBI, as compared with orthopedic injuries (OI). BRIEF ratings, measures of family functioning—including the Family Burden of Injury Interview (FBII) and Family Assessment Device (FAD)—and the Brief Symptom Inventory (BSI) were completed by the parents. Neuropsychological testing included several measures of executive function. Scores on the BRIEF displayed a significant linear trend across groups, most with the largest deficits in executive functions reported in the severe TBI group. The BRIEF Behavioral Regulation and Metacognition Index scores were related consistently across all groups to the Consonant Trigrams test, a test of working memory. The BRIEF Index scores also predicted parent psychological distress (BSI) and perceived family burden (FBII), in the TBI and OI groups. In contrast, general family functioning as measured by the FAD was related to BRIEF scores only in the TBI groups. These findings demonstrate the relation between executive function, as measured by the BRIEF, as well as parent and family stress. Among families of children with TBI, general family functioning may be particularly stressed by the injured child's executive dysfunction. An ecologically valid measure of executive function, such as the BRIEF, reveals this relation in ways that performance-based tests do not.

Several points regarding the ecological validity of executive function are highlighted by Armstrong et al.'s study. First, injury severity was associated with everyday manifestations of executive function. This finding extends the findings of other authors who have used only performance-based tests (e.g., Levin et al., 1994) in relating injury severity to neuropsychological outcome. It also differs from the findings of Dennis et al. (2001), who did not find injury severity to be related to parent ratings of attentional control or social–behavioral regulation. Second, a traditional performance-based test of working memory (i.e., Consonant Trigrams) was associated with an everyday manifestation of executive dysfunction in the BRIEF.

Studies such as Armstrong et al. (2001) with the BRIEF and Dennis et al. (2001) with specific behavior ratings highlight the utility of real-world behavioral anchors with which traditional neuropsychological test performances and injury variables can be related. Test-based and behavior rating-based outcomes provide not only information on the specific components of executive function but also seeks to identify their real-world functional manifestations. Neuropsychological dysfunction on a test should not be the end goal in itself but instead highlight specific ways in which the child manifests problems with executive function. Finally, Armstong et al. highlight the role of the family context in terms of its importance in the child's executive function. Ecologically valid measurement of executive function, as provided by the BRIEF, allows examination of critical, family-contextual determinants. Such an assessment model ties the everyday executive function outcome of the child with TBI into a broader systemic context and begins to define the foci for active intervention within the child and the caretaking system.

SUMMARY

Executive dysfunction is a common outcome in children who have sustained TBI. Appropriate assessment of executive functions is critical to plan necessary interventions. Because executive functions are a complex, environmentally sensitive set of interrelated processes, their assessment challenges our traditional testing methodologies. Ecological validity has become an increasingly important focus in neuropsychological assessment with a number of authors articulating the critical issues (Cripe, 1996; Silver, 2000). This article highlights two important issues—veridicality and verisimilitude—that neuropsychological measures must consider. Tests can vary in the degree to which they are highly structured and controlled, such as in a laboratory or clinical setting versus a less-structured real-world setting. They can also vary in terms of their face and content validity, as well as in their ability to predict real-world behavior. Given the nature of the executive functions with their inherent focus on managing and coordinating cognitive and behavioral activities in response to real-world demands, ecological validity is particularly important in their assessment. The BRIEF was explicitly developed with an eye to these issues of ecological validity. Within the various theoretical domains described by others, items tapping specific, everyday behaviors were generated to capture the real-world behavioral manifestations of executive dysfunction. In addition to meeting traditional standards of reliability and validity, the BRIEF also demonstrates ecological validity with its inherent focus on the actual, everyday behaviors of children.

Returning to TBI, or for that matter any complex disorder involving the executive functions, we submit that an ecologically valid approach to the assessment of these self-control functions is critical to provide appropriate intervention. The work by Armstrong et al. (2001) and Dennis et al. (2001) provide an instructive example toward this end. These studies highlight a multilevel approach to understanding neuropsychological outcome in TBI. Traditional test-based measures of executive function are given to tap specific components of executive function such as working memory, inhibition, and organization. One might describe this level as the component or molecular level. Armstrong et al. defined the child's real-world behavioral manifestation of executive dysfunction via the BRIEF. This characterizes the molar level of function in the child, describing the ways that the specific components might play out in terms of everyday behaviors. Finally, the environmental system factors are revealed including the family structure and resources and parent-coping skills. These are key, facilitating factors necessary for full ecologically sensitive interventions directed at the molar and molecular levels of the child's behaviors. In this model, the ecologically valid assessment of executive dysfunction provides an important bridge toward understanding how the component-level (i.e., test-based) deficits impact on the child's everyday adaptive functioning. The definition of real-world behaviors also provides actual behaviors, situations, or both, toward which interventions may be directed.

We advocate for an ecologically valid model of neuropsychological assessment that explicitly incorporates at least three levels of information—(a) specific process components typically defined by clinical tests, (b) real-world behavioral manifestations of the specific cognitive processes, and (c) the environmental systems factors that impact on the child's function. An assessment approach that balances these three elements would incorporate the traditional psychometric qualities of reliability and validity while also providing strong ecological validity. Such a comprehensive approach would better guide intervention planning and monitoring—the ultimate goal of good neuropsychological assessment.

REFERENCES

Achenbach, T. (1991). *Manual for the Child Behavior Checklist/4–18 and 1991 profile*. Burlington, VT: University of Vermont Department of Psychiatry.

Achenbach, T., McConaughy, S., & Howell, C. (1987). Child/adolescent behavioral and emotional problems: Implications of cross-informant correlations for situational specificity. *Psychological Bulletin, 101*, 213–232.

Ackerly, S. S. (1964). A case of perinatal bilateral frontal lobe defect observed for thirty years. In J. M. Warren & K. Akert (Eds.), *The Frontal Granular Cortex and Behavior*. New York: McGraw-Hill.

Anderson, V. (1998). Assessing executive functions in children: Biological, psychological and developmental considerations. *Neuropsychological Rehabilitation, 8*, 319–349.

Anderson, V., Catroppa, C., Rosenfeld, J., Haritou, F., & Morse, S. A. (2000). Recovery of memory function following traumatic brain injury in pre-school children. *Brain Injury, 14,* 679–692.

Armstrong, K., Mangeot, S., Colvin, A., Yeates, K. O., & Taylor, H. G. (2001). *Long-term executive deficits in children with traumatic brain injuries.* Unpublished manuscript.

Asarnow, R. F., Satz, P., Light, R., & Neumann, E. (1991). Behavior problems and adaptive functioning in children with mild and severe closed head injury. *Journal of Pediatric Psychology, 16,* 543–555.

Barkley, R. (1997). *ADHD and the Nature of Self-Control.* New York: Guilford.

Barkley, R. A. (2000). Genetics of childhood disorders: XVII. ADHD, Part 1: The executive functions and ADHD. *Journal of American Academy of Child and Adolescent Psychiatry, 39,* 1064–1068.

Bayless, J. D., Varney, N. R., & Roberts, R. J. (1989). Tinker Toy Test performance and vocational outcome in patients with closed-head injuries. *Journal of Clinical and Experimental Neuropsychology, 11,* 913–917.

Bernstein, J. H., & Waber, D. P. (1990). Developmental neuropsychological assessment: The systemic approach. In A. A. Boulton, G. B. Baker, & M. Hiscock (Eds.), *Neuromethods: Vol. 17 Neuropsychology.* Clifton, NJ: Humana.

Brown, T. E. (1999). Does ADHD Diagnosis require impulsivity-hyperactivity?: A response to Gordon & Barkley. *ADHD Report, 7,* 1–7.

Brunswick, E. (1955). Symposium of the probability approach in psychology: Representative design and probabilistic theory in a functional psychology. *Psychological Review, 62,* 193–217.

Burgess, P. W. (1997). Theory and methodology in executive function and research. In P. Rabbitt (Ed.), *Methodology of frontal and executive function* (pp. 81–116). Hove, UK: Psychology.

Burgess, P. W., Alderman, N., Evans, J., Emslie, H., & Wilson, B. A. (1998). The ecological validity of tests of executive function. *Journal of the International Neuropsychological Society, 4,* 547–558.

Burgess, P. W., Alderman, N., Wilson, B. A., Evans, J. J., & Emslie, H. (1996). The Dysexecutive Questionnaire. In B. A. Wilson, N. Alderman, P. W. Burgess, H. Emslie, & J. J. Evans (Eds.), *Behavioral assessment of the dysexecutive syndrome.* Edmunds, England: Thames Valley Test Company.

Conners, C. K. (1989). *Manual for Conners' Rating Scales.* North Tonawanda, NY: Multi-Health Systems.

Cripe, Lloyd I. (1996). The ecological validity of executive function testing. In R. J. Sbordone & C. J. Long (Eds.), *Ecological validity of neuropsychological testing* (pp. 171–202). Delray Beach, FL: St. Lucie.

Cronbach, L. J. (1951). Coefficient alpha and the internal structure of tests. *Psychometrika, 16,* 297–334.

Denckla, M. B. (1989). Executive function, the overlap zone between attention deficit hyperactivity disorder and learning disabilities. *International Pediatrics, 4,* 155–160.

Denckla, M. B. (1994). Measurement of executive function. In G. R. Lyon (Ed.), *Frames of reference for the assessment of learning disabilities: New views on measurement issues* (pp. 117–142). Baltimore: Brookes.

Denckla, M. B. (1996). A theory and model of executive function: A neuropsychological perspective. In G. R. Lyon & N. A. Krasnegor (Eds.), *Attention, memory and executive function* (pp. 263–278). Baltimore: Brookes.

Dennis, M. (1991). Frontal lobe function in childhood and adolescence: A heuristic for assessing attention regulation, executive control, and the intentional states important for social discourse. *Developmental Neuropsychology, 7,* 327–358.

Dennis, M. (2000). Childhood medical disorders and cognitive impairment: Biological risk, time, development, and reserve. In K. O. Yeates, M. D. Ris, & H. G. Taylor (Eds.), *Pediatric neuropsychology: Research, theory and practice* (pp. 3–22). New York: Guilford.

Dennis, M., Guger, S., Roncadin, C., Barnes, M., & Schachar, R. (2001). Attentional-inhibitory and social-behavioral regulation after childhood closed head injury: Do biological, developmental, and recovery variables predict outcome? *Journal of the International Neuropsychological Society, 7,* 683–692.

Dennis, M., Barnes, M. A., Donnelly, R. E., Wilkinson, M., & Humphreys, R. P. (1996). Appraising and managing knowledge: Metacognitive skills after childhood head injury. *Developmental Neuropsychology, 12,* 77–103.

Dunn, E. J., Searight, H. R., Grisso, T., Margolis, R. B., & Gibbons, J. L. (1990). The relation of the Halstead-Reitan Neuropsychological Battery to functional daily living skills in geriatric patients. *Archives of Clinical Neuropsychology, 5,* 103–117.

Eslinger, P. J. (1998). Neurological and neuropsychological bases of empathy. *European Neurology, 39,* 193–199.

Eslinger, P. J., Biddle, K. R., & Grattan, L. M. (1997). Cognitive and Social development in children with prefrontal cortex lesions. In N. A. Krasnegor, G. R. Lyon, & P. S. Goldman-Rakic (Eds.), *Development of the prefrontal cortex: Evolution, Neurobiology and Behavior* (pp. 295–335). Baltimore: Brookes.

Eslinger, P. J., & Damasio, A. R. (1985). Severe disturbance of higher cognition after bilateral frontal lobe ablation. *Neurology, 35,* 1731–1741.

Eslinger, P. J., & Grattan L. M. (1991). Perspectives on the developmental consequences of early frontal lobe damage: Introduction. *Developmental Neuropsychology, 7,* 257–260.

Ewing-Cobbs, L., Prasad, M., Fletcher, J. M., Levin, H. S., Miner, M. E., & Eisenberg, H. M. (1998). Attention after pediatric traumatic brain injury: A multidimensional assessment. *Child Neuropsychology, 4,* 35–48.

Fletcher, J. M. Ewing-Cobbs, L., Miner, M. E., Levin, H. S., & Eisenberg, H. (1990). Behavioral changes after closed head injury in children. *Journal of Consulting and Clinical Psychology, 58,* 93–98.

Franzen, M. D., & Wilhelm, K. L. (1996). Conceptual foundations of ecological validity in neuropsychological assessment. In R. J. Sbordone & C. J. Long (Eds.), *Ecological validity of neuropsychological testing* (pp. 91–112). Boca Raton, FL: St. Lucie.

Fuster, J. M. (1985). The prefrontal cortex, mediator of cross-temporal contingencies. *Human Neurobiology, 4,* 169–179.

Fuster, J. M. (1989). *The prefrontal cortex: Anatomy, physiology, and neurophysiology of the frontal lobe.* New York: Raven.

Gioia, G. A., & Isquith, P. K. (in press). Executive function and ADHD: Exploration through children's everyday behaviors. *Clinical Neuropsychological Assessment.*

Gioia, G. A., Isquith, P. K., & Guy, S. C. (1998). The regulatory role of executive control processes in children's behavioral, social, and emotional functioning. *Journal of Neuropsychiatry and Clinical Neurosciences, 9,* 663.

Gioia, G. A., Isquith, P. K., Guy, S. C., & Kenworthy, L. (2000). *Behavior Rating Inventory of Executive Function.* Odessa, FL: Psychological Assessment Resources.

Goldberg, E., & Podell, K. (2000). Adaptive decision making, ecological validity, and the frontal lobes. *Journal of Clinical and Experimental Neuropsychology, 22,* 56–68.

Goldman-Rakic, P. (1987). Circuitry of primate prefrontal cortex and regulation of behavior by representational memory. In F. Plum (Ed.), *Handbook of Physiology: The Nervous System* (pp. 373–417). NY: Oxford University Press.

Goulden, L. G., Silver, C. H., Harward, H. S., & Levin, H. S. (1997). Utility of the Children's Executive Functions Scale in childhood brain injury. *Archives of Clinical Neuropsychology, 12,* 326.

Hart, T., & Hayden, M. D. (1986). The ecological validity of neuropsychological assessment and remediation. In B. P. Uzzell & Y. Gross (Eds.), *Clinical Neuropsychology of Intervention* (pp. 21–50). Boston: Martinus Nijhoff.

Hartlage, L. C., & Templer, D. I. (1996). Ecological issues in child neuropsychological assessment. In R. J. Sbordone & C. J. Long (Eds.), *Ecological validity of neuropsychological testing* (pp. 301–313). New York: St. Lucie.

Heaton, R., Chelune, G., Talley, J., Kay, G., & Curtiss, G. (1993). *Wisconsin Card Sorting Test Manual.* Odessa, FL: Psychological Assessment Resources.

Isquith, P. K., & Gioia, G. A. (1999). The nature of executive functioning in ADHD. *Clinical Neuropsychologist, 13,* 227.

Isquith, P. K., & Gioia, G. A. (2000). Brief predictions of ADHD: Clinical utility of the Behavior Rating Inventory of Executive Function for detecting ADHD subtypes in children. *Archives of Clinical Neuropsychology, 15,* 780–781.

Janusz, J., Ahluvalia, T., & Gioia, G. A. (2001). *The relationship between executive function and adaptive behavior.* Unpublished manuscript.

Kaplan, E. (1988). A process approach to neuropsychological assessment. In T. Boll & B. K. Bryant (Eds.), *Clinical neuropsychology and brain function: Research, measurement and practice* (pp. 125–167). Washington, DC: American Psychological Association.

Kelly, T. P. (2000). The development of executive function in school-aged children. *Clinical Neuropsychological Assessment, 1,* 38–55.

Kibby, M. Y., Schmitter-Edgecombe, M., & Long, C. J. (1998). Ecological validity of neuropsychological tests: Focus on the California Verbal Learning Test and the Wisconsin Card Sorting Test. *Archives of Clinical Neuropsychology, 13,* 523–534.

Levin, H. S., Culhane, K. A., Hartmann, J., Evankovich, K., Mattson, A. J., Harward, H., et al. (1991). Developmental changes in performance on tests of purported frontal lobe functioning. *Developmental Neuropsychology, 7,* 377–395.

Levin, H. S., Culhane, K. A., Mendelsohn, E., Lilly, M. A., Bruce, D., Fletcher, J., et al. (1993). Cognition in relation to magnetic resonance imaging in head-injured children and adolescents. *Archives of Neurology, 50,* 897–905.

Levin, H. S., Fletcher, J. M., Kufera, J. A., Harward, H., Lilly, M. A., Mendelsohn, D., et al. (1996). Dimensions of cognition measured by the Tower of London and other cognitive tasks in head-injured children and adolescents. *Developmental Neuropsychology, 12,* 17–34.

Levin, H. S., Mendelsohn, D., Lily, M. A., Fletcher, J. M., Culhane, K. A., Chapman, S. B., et al. (1994). Tower of London performance in relation to magnetic resonance imaging following closed head injury in children. *Neuropsychology, 8,* 171–179.

Lezak, M. D. (1982). The problem of assessing executive functions. *International Journal of Psychology, 17,* 281–297.

Lezak, M. (1995). *Neuropsychological assessment* (3rd ed.). New York: Oxford University Press.

Long, C. J. (1996). Neuropsychological tests: A look at our past and the impact that ecological issues may have on our future. In R. J. Sbordone & C. J. Long (Eds.), *Ecological validity of neuropsychological testing* (pp. 1–14). Boca Raton, FL: St. Lucie.

Lysaker, P., Bell, M., & Bean-Goulet, J. (1995). Wisconsin Card Sorting Test and work performance in schizophrenia. *Psychiatry Research, 56,* 45–51.

Mahone, E. M., Koth, C. W., Cutting, L., Singer, H. S., & Denckla, M. B. (2001). Executive function in fluency and recall measures among children with Tourette syndrome or ADHD. *Journal of the International Neuropsychological Society, 7,* 102–111.

Manly, T., Robertson, I. H., Anderson, V., & Nimmo-Smith, I. (1999). *Test of Everyday Attention for Children.* Bury St. Edmunds, UK: Thames Valley Test Company Limited.

Marlowe, W. (1992). The impact of right prefrontal lesion on the developing brain. *Brain and Cognition, 20,* 205–213.

Molho, C. E., & Silver, C. H. (1997). An investigation of the Children's Executive functions Scale. *Archives of Clinical Neuropsychology, 12,* 370.

Pennington, B. F., & Ozonoff, S. (1996). Executive functions and developmental psychopathology. *Journal of Child Psychology and Psychiatry, 37,* 51–87.

Pennington, B. F., Bennetto, L., McAleer, O. K., & Roberts, R. J. (1996). Executive functions and working memory: Theoretical and measurement issues. In G. R. Lyon & N. A. Krasnegor (Eds.), *Attention, memory and executive function*. Baltimore: Brookes.

Rabbitt, P. (1997). Introduction: Methodologies and models in the study of executive function. In P. Rabbitt (Ed.), *Methodology of frontal executive function* (pp. 1–38). East Sussex, UK: Psychology.

Rabin, L. (2001). *Test usage patterns and perceived ecological utility of neuropsychological assessment techniques: A survey of North American clinical neuropsychologists*. Unpublished doctoral dissertation, Oxford University.

Reynolds, C. R., & Kamphaus, R. W. (1994). *Behavior Assessment System for Children*. Circle Pines, MN: American Guidance Service.

Roberts, M. A., Franzen, K. M., Furuseth, A., & Fuller, L. (1995). A developmental study of the Tinker Toy® Test: Normative and clinical observations. *Applied Neuropsychology, 2,* 161–166.

Sbordone, R. J. (1996). Ecological validity: Some critical issues for the neuropsychologist. In R. J. Sbordone & C. J. Long (Eds.), *Ecological validity of neuropsychological testing* (pp. 91–112). Boca Raton, FL: St. Lucie.

Scheibel, R. S., & Levin, H. S. (1997). Frontal lobe dysfunction following closed head injury in children: Findings from neuropsychology and brain injury. In N. A. Krasnegor, G. R. Lyon, & P. S. Goldman-Rakic (Eds.), *Development of the prefrontal cortex: Evolution, neurobiology and behavior*. Baltimore: Brookes.

Shallice, T., & Burgess, P. W. (1991). Deficits in strategy application following frontal lobe damage in man. *Brain, 114,* 727–741.

Silver, C. (2000). Ecological validity in neuropsychological assessment in childhood traumatic brain injury. *Journal of Head Trauma Rehabilitation, 15,* 973–988.

Sparrow, S. S., Balla, D. A., & Cicchetti, Domenic V. (1984). *Vineland Adaptive Behavior Scales*. Circle Pines, MN: American Guidance Service.

Stuss, D. T., & Benson, D. F. (1986). *The frontal lobes*. New York: Raven.

Stuss, D. T., & Buckle, L. (1992). Traumatic brain injury: Neuropsychological deficits and evaluation at different stages of recovery and in different pathologic subtypes. *Journal of Head Trauma Rehabilitation, 7,* 40–49.

Taylor, H. G., Yeates, K. O., Wade, S. L., Drotar, D., Klein, S. K., & Stancin, T. (1999). Influences on first-year recovery from traumatic brain injury in children. *Neuropsychology, 13,* 76–89.

Taylor, H. G., Yeates, K. O., Wade, S. L., Drotar, D., Stancin, T., & Burant, C. (2001). Bidirectional child-family influences on outcomes of traumatic brain injury in children. *Journal of the International Neuropsychological Society, 7,* 755–767.

Wade, S. L., Borawski, E. A., Taylor, H. G., Drotar, D. Yeates, K. O., & Stancin, T. (2001). The relationship of caregiver coping to family outcomes during the initial year following pediatric traumatic injury. *Journal of Consulting & Clinical Psychology, 69,* 406–415.

Welsh, M. C., & Pennington, B. F. (1988). Assessing frontal lobe functioning in children: Views from developmental psychology. *Developmental Neuropsychology, 4,* 199–230.

Welsh, M. C., Pennington, B. F., & Grossier, D. B. (1991). A normative-developmental study of executive function: A window on prefrontal function in children. *Developmental Neuropsychology, 7,* 131–149.

Wilson, B. A., Evans, J. J., Emslie, H., Alderman, N., & Burgess, P. (1998). The development of an ecologically valid test for assessing patients with a dysexecutive syndrome. *Neuropsychological Rehabilitation, 8,* 213–228.

Yeates, K. O., Taylor, H. G., Drotar, D., Wade, S., Stancin, T., & Klein, S. (1997). Preinjury family environment as a determinant of recovery from traumatic brain injury in school-age children. *Journal of the International Neuropsychological Society, 3,* 617–630.

Ylvisaker, M. (Ed.). (1998). *Traumatic brain injury rehabilitation: Children and adolescents* (2nd ed.). Boston: Butterworth-Heinemann.

Ylvisaker, M., & Feeney, T. J. (1998). *Collaborative brain injury intervention: Positive Everyday Routines*. San Diego, CA: Singular Publishing Group.

Ylvisaker, M., & Gioia, G. A. (1998). Cognitive assessment. In M. Ylvisaker (Ed.), *Traumatic brain injury rehabilitation: Children and adolescents* (2nd ed.). Boston: Butterworth-Heinemann.

Ylvisaker, M. Szekeres, S., & Hartwick, P. (1992). Cognitive rehabilitation following Traumatic brain injury in children. In M. G. Tramontana & S. R. Hooper (Eds.), *Advances in child neuropsychology* (pp. 168–218). New York: Springer.

DEVELOPMENTAL NEUROPSYCHOLOGY, 25(1&2), 159–177

Attention Deficit Hyperactivity Disorder in Children and Adolescents Following Traumatic Brain Injury

Jeffrey E. Max

Department of Psychiatry
University of California, San Diego
Children's Hospital and Health Center, San Diego

Amy E. Lansing

Veterans Hospital, San Diego
Children's Hospital and Health Center, San Diego

Sharon L. Koele

Department of Psychiatry
University of Iowa

Carlos S. Castillo

Cedar Centre
Cedar Rapids, Iowa

Hirokazu Bokura

Yasugi Daiichi Hospital
Department of Neurology
Shimane, Japan

Russell Schachar

Brain and Behavior Program, Research Institute
Hospital for Sick Children
Toronto, Ontario, Canada

Requests for reprints should be sent to Jeffrey E. Max, Children's Hospital and Health Center, 3020 Children's Way, MC 5033, San Diego, CA 92123–4282. E-mail: jmax@ucsd.edu

Nicole Collings and Kathryn E. Williams

Children's Hospital and Health Center, San Diego

To better characterize pediatric psychopathology after neurological insult, secondary attention deficit hyperactivity disorder (SADHD)—or ADHD that develops after traumatic brain injury (TBI)—and its clinical and neuroimaging correlates were investigated. Outcome data were available for 118 children, ages 5 through 14 at the time of hospitalization following TBI (severe TBI $n = 37$; mild–moderate TBI $n = 57$) and orthopedic injury ($n = 24$). Standardized psychiatric, adaptive functioning, cognitive functioning, family functioning, and family psychiatric history assessments were conducted on all participants. Severity of injury and neuroimaging lesion assessments were conducted on TBI participants only. The diagnosis of SADHD was mutually exclusive with preinjury ADHD, which occurred in 13 of 94 TBI participants and 4 of 24 orthopedic injury participants. SADHD occurred in 13 of 34 eligible participants with severe TBI but resolved in 4 of 13 of these participants. SADHD also occurred in 1 of 8 eligible moderate TBI participants, only in the presence of preinjury ADHD traits and 3 of 39 of eligible mild TBI cases. SADHD occurred in 1 of 20 of eligible participants with orthopedic injury without any brain injury. SADHD was significantly associated with TBI severity recorded by categorical and dimensional measures, intellectual and adaptive functioning deficits, and personality change due to TBI, but not with lesion area or location. These results suggest that SADHD is a clinically important syndrome after severe TBI in children and adolescents.

Attention deficit hyperactivity disorder (ADHD) and childhood traumatic brain injury (TBI) are both major public health problems. ADHD is a psychiatric disorder that affects up to 6% of children (Szatmari, Offord, & Boyle, 1989) and there are 100,000 children under the age of 15 years admitted to hospitals annually for TBI in the United States (Kraus, Fife, & Conroy, 1987). Understanding the relation between ADHD and TBI in children and adolescents is critically important for clinicians, researchers, and the civil justice system. To date, this relation has been investigated in a preliminary fashion. Our goal in this article is to use psychiatric, family, cognitive, and neuroimaging data to refine the understanding of the relation between TBI and ADHD.

PREINJURY ADHD AND CHILDHOOD TBI

Preinjury ADHD may confound studies of postinjury ADHD. Specifically, there is evidence to support a hypothesis of hyperactivity and attention deficits among children whose behavior may have been a factor in the occurrence of an injury compared with injured children whose behavior was not a factor in the injury

(Pless, Taylor, & Arsenault, 1995). However, data on the rate of preinjury ADHD in children who sustain a TBI are scant. There are only two published prospective studies of consecutively admitted children with TBI that have used standardized psychiatric interviews to retrospectively assess preinjury psychiatric disorders at the earliest feasible postinjury opportunity (Brown, Chadwick, Shaffer, Rutter, & Traub, 1981; Max, Robin, et al., 1997). Only one of these studies (Max, Robin, et al., 1997) measured preinjury ADHD and found a rate of 10%. A retrospective study of consecutively admitted participants with severe TBI found a preinjury rate of 13% (Max, Koele, et al., 1998). Bloom et al. (2001) sampled 46 consecutively admitted participants in a prospective study of TBI only if a developmental screen for psychiatric disorders, including ADHD, was negative. A standardized psychiatric interview assessment conducted at least 1 year postinjury concluded that the onset of ADHD occurred in 10 of 46 (22%) participants *before* the injury.

There are also preinjury ADHD data, based on standardized psychiatric interviews, from two studies of referred samples. First, a prospective study found that 20% (19 of 99) of moderate–severe TBI participants referred to a rehabilitation center had preinjury ADHD (Gerring et al., 1998). Second, a retrospective study of mild-to-severe TBI participants referred to a pediatric brain injury clinic found that 20% (10 of 50) of participants had preinjury ADHD (Max, Lindgren, et al., 1997).

POSTINJURY ADHD AND CHILDHOOD TBI

Data on the rate of postinjury ADHD (hereafter referred to as secondary ADHD or SADHD) in children who sustained a TBI are also limited. In fact, *there are no data linking the presence of SADHD to severity of TBI.* The occurrence of SADHD or "hyperkinetic syndrome" diagnosed by structured psychiatric interviews varied from 8% to 53% (Bloom et al., 2001; Brown et al., 1981; Gerring et al., 1998; Max, Koele, et al., 1998; Max, Lindgren, et al., 1998; Max, Robin, et al., 1997). This extremely wide range was related to study design (prospective or retrospective, consecutive hospital admissions, or referred–convenience samples), psychiatric interview used (specific screening for ADHD), and participant characteristics (range of TBI severity and proportion of mild, moderate, and severe TBI participants). The studies either did not analyze the relation between SADHD and severity of injury (Brown et al., 1981; Max, Koele, et al., 1998; Max, Robin, et al., 1997), or no relation was found because of a restricted range of severity studied (Gerring et al., 1998) and because of the referred or convenience samples studied (Bloom et al., 2001; Max, Lindgren, et al., 1998). The course of SADHD after the injury has not been systematically reported and little is known about the course of preexisting ADHD after the injury in TBI participants (Gerring et al., 1998).

A link between SADHD or "hyperkinetic" syndrome and the diagnosis of personality change due to TBI (formerly referred to as frontal lobe syndrome) characterized by disinhibition and affective instability has been suggested (Brown et al., 1981; Gerring et al., 1998; Max et al., 2000). Gerring and colleagues (1998) found participants with SADHD had greater posttraumatic affective lability, aggression, comorbidity, and overall more disability than children who did not develop SADHD. These investigators also found that deep brain lesions, including those of thalamus, right putamen, and "basal ganglia," were associated with SADHD (Gerring et al., 2000; Herskovits et al., 1999). A retrospective study of a pediatric brain injury clinic referred sample found that there were no variables (including impaired family functioning, family psychiatric history, and severity of injury) that correlated significantly with SADHD (Max, Lindgren, et al., 1998).

The aforementioned data suggest that ADHD does occur before and after TBI in childhood. What is unclear, however, is the postinjury diagnostic stability and level of impairment of children with SADHD, as well as the relation of SADHD with injury and psychosocial variables. We specifically aimed to elucidate these issues. We hypothesized that SADHD would be significantly correlated with increasing severity of injury because of studies showing increased hyperactive–impulsive and inattentive symptomatology studied as dimensional variables rather than a categorical diagnosis in prospective studies of TBI participants with a full range of injury severity (Knights et al., 1991; Max, Arndt, et al., 1998). We hypothesized further that as a consequence the syndrome would be significantly associated with intellectual and adaptive functioning deficits. We expected that SADHD would be related to personality change due to TBI. Finally, we hypothesized that frontostriatal lesion location and lesion area would be significantly associated with SADHD (Gerring et al., 2000; Herskovitz et al., 1999). Although the data in this report are derived from two of our previously published studies (Max, Koele, et al., 1998; Max, Robin, et al., 1997), we have combined the data from these studies to increase the power of the analyses and shed light on the course and correlates of the diagnosis of SADHD.

METHOD

Participants

The participants were participants from two nonoverlapping studies of TBI in children and adolescents conducted between 1992 and 1997 (Max, Koele, et al., 1998; Max, Robin, et al., 1997). We have previously reported analyses on attention deficit hyperactivity *symptoms* from one of these studies (Max, Arndt, et al., 1998).

Study 1

The first study was *prospective,* in which all participants suffered either a mild, moderate, or severe TBI (see definitions under neurological assessment) and were consecutively admitted between 1992 and 1994 (Max, Robin, et al., 1997). Recruitment occurred at a university hospital, two regional hospitals, and a community hospital. Comprehensive psychiatric, family, and adaptive functioning assessments were conducted at "baseline" ($M = 14.8$ days, $SD = 13.1$ days after injury) to assess preinjury functioning and the assessments were repeated 3, 6, 12, and 24 months after TBI. Cognitive testing was also completed at each assessment except for the 6-month evaluation.

Inclusion criteria were as follows: (a) children aged 6 years through 14 years at time of mild, moderate, or severe closed head injury; (b) computed tomography (CT) scan of brain during hospitalization; (c) English as first language. Exclusion criteria were as follows: (a) posttraumatic amnesia (PTA) >3 months; (b) documented history of child abuse; (c) history of previous TBI involving at least one hospitalization longer than 1 night; (d) history of mental retardation; (e) other acquired or congenital central nervous system disorder; (f) preexisting acute or chronic serious illness.

A total of 87 TBI patients were hospitalized during the recruitment phase, 50 of whom were enrolled in the study (see Table 1 for enrollment and follow-up details). Severe TBI patients participated at a significantly higher rate (15 of 17) than the mild–moderate TBI patients (35 of 70; $p = .005$). The most common reason for nonparticipation was the parents of mild–moderate TBI children feeling confident that their child was back to baseline and that the scope of the study was therefore unwarranted. The study eligibility screen revealed there were no differences between participants and nonparticipants in terms of preinjury history of psychiatric–behavior disorder or psychiatric treatment–counseling (Max, Smith, et al., 1997).

Study 2

The second study was *retrospective* and involved a one-time assessment of participants at varied intervals from the time of injury (Max, Koele, et al., 1998). This study included consecutively hospitalized children and adolescents with severe TBI (admitted between 1988 and 1992), and an individually matched (regarding age, gender, ethnicity, socioeconomic status, and injury-to-assessment interval) group of mild TBI participants (see definitions of severity of TBI following), and a control group of children hospitalized for orthopedic injury. The severe TBI participants were recruited from the same university hospital and two regional hospitals as Study 1. Control participants were recruited from these hospitals, as well as from four community hospitals and another regional hospital.

Inclusion criteria were as follows: (a) children aged 5 through 14 years at the time of injury; (b) consecutive admissions following a severe TBI, and two discrete groups of their individual matches (children who suffered a mild TBI and children who suffered an orthopedic injury without a brain injury); and (c) CT scan of brain

TABLE 1

Preinjury and Secondary ADHD in Prospectively and Retrospectively Studied Injured Children

	No. Ss Enrolled/No. Ss Eligible (No. Ss With Follow-Up Data)	Preinjury ADHD	Course of Preinjury ADHD	SADHD	Course of SADHD
Study 1					
Total	50/87 total TBI enrolled (n = 46[a]; mild–moderate–severe TBI)	5/50		8/41	
Severe	15/17 severe TBI (n = 13[a])	0/15 severe TBI		7/13 severe TBI → →	Two resolved at 6 months One resolved at 18 months
Moderate	9/21 moderate TBI (n = 9)	1/9 moderate TBI →	One stable	1/8 moderate TBI →	One persisting at 24 months
Mild	26/49 mild TBI (n = 24)	4/26 mild TBI → →	Two stable Two resolved	0/20 mild TBI	
Study 2					
Total	72/77 total enrolled Ss (n = 72; mild–severe TBI, orthopedic)	12/72		10/60	
Severe	24/29 severe TBI (n = 24)	3/24 severe TBI → → →	One worse One improved One worse attention and improved hyperactivity	6/21 severe TBI →	All persisting (.5–3.3 years postinjury)
Mild	24/24 mild TBI (matched)	5/24 mild TBI →	Five stable	3/19 mild TBI →	All persisting (.8–3.3 years)
Orthopedic	24/24 orthopedic (matched)	4/24 orthopedic → →	Three stable One worse	1/20 orthopedic →	Persisted 3.1 years postinjury

Note. The denominator under the SADHD column denotes only participants who did not have preinjury ADHD and who also completed follow-up interviews. Ss = subjects; SADHD = secondary attention deficit hyperactivity disorder; TBI = traumatic brain injury.

[a]In addition to these Ss, there were preinjury psychiatric data available for one child who remained in a vegetative state.

164

during hospitalization for TBI participants. Exclusion criteria were as follows: (a) documented history of child maltreatment; (b) mild TBI patients with a clinical history of TBI before the index injury requiring at least an emergency room visit; (c) more than one mild TBI prior to the severe TBI for severe TBI participants; (d) orthopedic injury participants with any clinical history of TBI; (e) history of mental retardation; (f) other acquired or congenital central nervous system disorder; (g) quadriplegia; (h) patients unable to participate in a semistructured interview (e.g., persistent vegetative state); and (i) residence >300 miles away.

Chart review revealed 29 eligible patients with severe TBI, 24 (82.4%) of whom, along with their mild TBI matches and orthopedic injury matches, participated in the study (see Table 1 for details). Three eligible severe TBI participants were unreachable and two refused.

The inclusion and exclusion criteria for Study 1 and Study 2 were comparable, except that moderate TBI participants were included only in Study 1, orthopedic participants were included only in the study 2, and several children aged 5 at the time of TBI were included in Study 2. The latter difference contributed to the significantly younger age at injury (8.7 ± 3.1 versus 10.4 ± 2.5 years; $p = .007$) and age at assessment (10.9 ± 3.5 versus 12.3 ± 2.5 years; $p < .03$) in children from Study 2. The groups did not differ in the interval from injury to assessment or socioeconomic status. Table 2 illustrates the demographics of all Study 1 and Study 2 participants. After presenting a complete description of the study to the participants, written informed consent was obtained from parents–guardians and assent was obtained from the children. Based on screening in both of the studies, no significant differences were found

TABLE 2
Demographic Factors

	All TBI Participants[a]	Mild–Moderate TBI Participants[b]	Severe TBI Participants[c]	Orthopedic Participants[a]	Significance
Mean age at injury (SD)	9.53 (2.92)	9.30 (2.66)	9.62 (3.36)	8.81 (3.29)	ns
Mean age at last assessment (SD)	11.61 (3.09)	11.60 (2.76)	11.64 (3.58)	10.92 (3.37)	ns
Mean injury to assessment (SD)	2.07 (0.77)	2.13 (0.79)	1.98 (0.74)	2.07 (1.10)	ns
Boys n (%)	58 (62)	33 (58)	25 (68)	18 (75)	ns
White n (%)	92 (98)	57 (100)	35 (95)	23 (96)	ns
Mean SES (SD)	2.77 (1.07)	2.63 (1.10)	2.97 (1.01)	2.46 (0.83)	ns

Note. Socioeconomic class assessment was accomplished through the Four Factor Index (Hollingshead, 1975). Significance refers to the comparison between the severe versus the mild–moderate groups tested by independent sample t tests or chi-square tests. TBI = traumatic brain injury; SES = socioeconomic status.
[a]$n = 94$. [b]$n = 57$. [c]$n = 37$. [d]$n = 24$.

regarding age, gender, ethnicity, and SES when comparing the nonparticipating plus "drop-out" TBI participants (mild–moderate $n = 37$, severe $n = 8$) with their respective severity-class participating counterparts (Table 1).

Measures

Neurological assessments.   Severity of TBI classification depended on the lowest postresuscitation score on the Glasgow Coma Scale (GCS; Teasdale & Jennett, 1974), which was recorded from clinical notes. The GCS is the standard measure of severity of brain injury in the acute stage of injury. Severe TBI was defined by a lowest postresuscitation GCS score ≤8. Moderate injury was defined by a lowest postresuscitation GCS score of 9–12 or a score of 13–15 with an intracranial lesion or with a depressed skull fracture seen on the initial CT scan (Williams, Levin, & Eisenberg, 1990). Mild injury was defined by a lowest postresuscitation GCS score of 13 to 15, with or without a linear skull fracture. Duration of impaired consciousness was defined as the time from injury to the attainment of a score of 6 (ability to follow commands) on the motor subscale of the GCS based on clinical notes.

The initial CT scans were analyzed independently by a pediatric radiologist and by a pediatric neuroradiologist and then a consensus was reached by discussion in the case of discrepancies. Lesion location was determined using a two-dimensional template method (Damasio & Damasio, 1989) and lesion area was calculated after digitization (Max, Arndt, et al., 1998).

Psychiatric measures.   Psychiatric diagnoses were derived by conducting the Schedule for Affective Disorders and Schizophrenia for School-Age Children (K–SADS; Chambers et al., 1985; Orvaschel, Puig-Antich, Chamber, Tabrizi, & Johnson, 1982). *Diagnostic and Statistical Manual* (3rd ed. rev. [*DSM–III–R*], American Psychiatric Association, 1987) criteria were used. We waived the age of onset criterion for ADHD to identify SADHD as it occurred in all children, including those ≥7 years. This instrument has been shown to provide excellent reliability and accuracy for the diagnosis of ADHD in circumstances in which diagnoses at the most recent testing are used as retrospective predictors of diagnoses made 1 year earlier (Faraone, Biederman, & Milberger, 1995) and has excellent convergence validity with well-validated behavior checklist methodology regarding the diagnosis of ADHD (Biederman et al., 1993).

Another psychiatric semistructured interview, the Neuropsychiatric Rating Schedule (NPRS; Max, Castillo, Lindgren, & Arndt, 1998) was used to identify symptoms and subtypes of personality change due to traumatic brain injury (PC) or organic personality syndrome (OPS).

All interviews were administered by Jeffrey E. Max, a board-certified child and adolescent psychiatrist, and almost all were videotaped. The clinician's assessment after integrating the parent's report, the participant's report, and the participant's clinical presentation was used in the analyses. Two other raters participated in interrater reliability studies. Sharon L. Koele, who was blind to specifics of the injury, viewed 9 Study 2 interviews and had perfect agreement (9 of 9) regarding the presence or absence of ADHD. Carlos S. Castillo viewed 10 Study 1 interviews and also had perfect agreement (10 of 10) regarding the presence or absence of ADHD.

Family psychiatric history. The Family History Research Diagnostic Criteria (Andreasen, Endicott, Spitzer, & Winokur, 1977) interview was conducted in most cases by Max and in other cases by two trained research assistants. Criteria were modified to conform with *DSM–III–R* criteria. Family ratings of status at the most recent research assessment were then summarized for first degree relatives on a 4-point scale ranging from 0 (*no psychiatric disorder*) to 3 (*psychiatric disorder with a history of inpatient treatment or incarceration in at least one first degree relative*; Max, Robin, et al., 1997) of increasing severity.

Family assessments. Global family functioning was assessed with the McMaster Structured Interview of Family Functioning. The interview is used to derive scores on the Clinical Rating Scale (CRS; Miller et al., 1994). The CRS comprises seven domains, including global family functioning, which are rated on a 7-point Likert scale ranging from 1 (*very poor*) to 7 (*superior*), in which lower scores indicate poorer function (see Table 5 note). The global family function rating at the most recent assessment was used in the analysis.

The Family of Life Events and Changes (FILE; McCubbin, Patterson, & Wilson, 1980) is a 71-item index of family stress with nine subscales and a total raw score. It was developed to measure the strain from life events and changes experienced by a family in the previous year. The score from the FILE completed by the primary caretaker at the latest assessment was used in the analyses.

Socioeconomic status. SES assessment was accomplished through the Four Factor Index (Hollingshead, 1975). Classification depends on scores derived from a formula involving both the mother's and father's educational levels and occupational levels. Scores of 1 through 5 were designated based on the range of scores within each of levels I–V. Higher scores indicated lower socioeconomic class.

Adaptive functioning measure. Adaptive functioning assessment was completed using the Vineland Adaptive Behavior Scale interview (Sparrow, Balla, & Cicchetti, 1984). This involved a semistructured interview conducted by a trained research assistant with the primary caretaker. Scores from the most recent research assessment were used in the analyses.

Intellectual function.   Intellectual functioning in Study 1 was assessed with subscales from the Wechsler Intelligence Scale for Children, Third Edition (WISC–III; Weschler, 1991). A prorated Full-Scale IQ (FIQ), derived from a prorated PIQ (Picture Arrangement, Block Design, and Coding subtests) and a prorated VIQ (Information and Similarities subtests) was obtained. The Wechsler Intelligence Scale for Children–Revised (WISC–R; Weschler, 1974) was used in Study 2. A prorated FIQ, derived from a prorated PIQ (Picture Arrangement, Block Design, and Coding subtests), and a prorated VIQ (Information, Similarities, Arithmetic, and Digit Span subtests) was obtained. The specific subtests in Study 2 were selected to parallel the Kaufman, Ishikuma, and Kaufman-Packer (1991) selection of WAIS–R short form subtests. We acknowledge that including digit span in the VIQ for the WISC–R in study 2 was suboptimal because this is not a standard part of the VIQ and because selection of subtests would be better if based on WISC data rather than WAIS–R data. The WISC–R scores from Study 2 were transformed into WISC–III equivalent scores using data from the test manual (Weschler, 1991), and these scores were used in the analyses. Scores from the most recent assessment were used in the analyses.

Statistical analysis.   We first describe the course and occurrence of preinjury ADHD and SADHD in TBI participants and orthopedic injury controls. Most of the formal statistical analyses that follow will be limited to TBI participants. The samples of participants with SADHD versus those without SADHD, and study participants versus nonparticipants were compared with independent sample *t* tests or chi-square analyses as appropriate. Nonparametric analyses were conducted when values were markedly skewed. Additionally, effect sizes were calculated for comparisons among severe TBI participants with and without SADHD because of smaller sample size.

RESULTS

Occurrence

Table 1 provides data on the occurrence and course of preinjury ADHD and SADHD in all participants, and demonstrates that preinjury ADHD was common across all injury categories. Examining the two studies, SADHD occurred frequently after severe TBI (13 of 34; even in participants with no preinjury ADHD symptoms), and less commonly after moderate TBI (1 of 8 cases, only with preinjury ADHD traits), and mild TBI (3 of 39). Further, SADHD occurred in the absence of TBI in 1 of 20 orthopedic injury children. The difference in the frequency of SADHD after severe TBI (13 of 34) compared with mild–moderate TBI (4 of 47) was significant ($p = .002$). Similarly, the difference in the frequency of

SADHD after severe TBI (13 of 34) compared with orthopedic participants (1 of 20) was significant ($p = .009$). There was no significant difference between the frequency of SADHD after mild–moderate TBI compared with orthopedic participants ($p > .52$).

Correlates of SADHD

Comorbidity.   Participants with transient SADHD and transient personality change due to TBI (PC) in addition to those with the persistent forms of these syndromes in children with mild, moderate, and severe TBI were investigated. Thirteen of 17 TBI participants with SADHD at any time (including 3 participants whose ADHD resolved) also had PC at some point after the injury, whereas 11 of 64 of children with no SADHD at any time had PC at some point after the injury, $\chi^2(1, N = 81) = 22.6, p < .0005$.

Injury factors.   Age at injury was not associated with SADHD when the analyses included all children with TBI (Table 3) or when children with severe TBI only were included (Table 4). Neither was gender significantly associated with SADHD: 11 of 52 boys versus 3 of 29 girls had SADHD in the full TBI cohort; 9 of 23 boys versus 1 of 11 girls had SADHD in the severe TBI cohort.

With injury severity considered as a continuous rather than a categorical variable, SADHD was again associated with greater severity of injury (lower GCS scores and longer duration of impaired consciousness, Table 3) when children with mild-to-severe TBI were analyzed.

We further investigated whether the relation of these injury factors and SADHD would persist when the sample was limited to children with severe TBI. Table 4

TABLE 3
Injury Factors and Persistent Secondary ADHD in Mild, Moderate, and Severe TBI

	No SADHD[a]		SADHD[b]		
	M	*SD*	*M*	*SD*	*Significance (p)*
Lowest postresuscitation GCS	11.1	4.3	7.6	4.8	.009
Hours of impaired consciousness[c]	114.7	361.2	288.4	567.6	.016
Lesion area[c] (cm²)	3.5	7.1	4.4	4.8	*ns*
Age at injury in years	9.6	3.1	8.9	2.6	*ns*
Age at assessment in years	11.7	3.2	11.2	2.7	*ns*

Note.   SADHD = secondary attention deficit hyperactivity disorder; TBI = traumatic brain injury; GCS = Glasgow Coma Scale score.
[a]$n = 67$. [b]$n = 14$. [c]Mann–Whitney U test.

TABLE 4
Injury Factors and Persistent Secondary ADHD in Severe TBI Participants

	No SADHD[a]		SADHD[b]			
	M	SD	M	SD	Significance (p)	Effect Size (d)
Lowest postresuscitation GCS	5.7	1.8	4.8	1.9	ns	.49
Hours of impaired consciousness[c]	319.2	553.6	403.8	643.1	ns	.14
Lesion area[c] (cm²)	8.6	9.6	5.2	4.8	ns	.45
Age at injury in years	10.0	3.5	8.5	2.7	ns	.48
Age at assessment in years	12.7	3.8	10.8	2.6	ns	.58

Note. Effect sizes (Cohen's *d*) of .20 to .49 are considered small, .50 to .79 are medium, and greater than .80 are large. SADHD = secondary attention deficit hyperactivity disorder; TBI = traumatic brain injury; GCS = Glasgow Coma Scale score.
[a]*n* = 24. [b]*n* = 10. [c]Mann–Whitney U test.

shows that within this narrower range of severity of injury, SADHD outcome was not associated with injury variables.

The initial CT scans identified cortical lesions in 30 of 37 severe TBI participants but no subcortical gray lesions. No specific lesion location (mesial frontal, lateral frontal, orbital frontal, lateral–superior temporal, mesial temporal, parietal, and occipital) correlated with the presence of SADHD in children with severe TBI. Neither did lesion area (Tables 3 and 4) correlate with the presence of SADHD.

Cognitive and adaptive function. Differences between children with SADHD and those without SADHD were observed in all tested domains of adaptive functioning and intellectual functioning (Table 5). Because it is well known that function in these domains is associated with severity of injury (Fay et al., 1994) and because we found that SADHD was associated with greater injury severity, we repeated the analyses in the severe TBI group only. Table 6 shows that the children with SADHD are still functioning significantly worse than children with no SADHD regarding adaptive and intellectual function.

Psychosocial variables. When children with mild-to-severe TBI were analyzed, *family function* was significantly worse in the SADHD group (Table 5). However, there were no significant differences regarding *socioeconomic status, family life events* (in the year preceding the latest assessment), *family psychiatric history, family history of ADHD, and lifetime preinjury psychiatric disorder in the child.* When only the severe TBI participants were analyzed, none of these

TABLE 5

Adaptive Behavior, Intellectual Function, and Psychosocial Adversity Variables in TBI Participants With and Without SADHD (Full Cohort)

	No SADHD[a]	n	SADHD[b]	n	Significance (p)
Timing of data collection in years postinjury (SD)	2.1 (.8)		2.3 (.9)		ns
Adaptive behavior composite SS mean (SD)	94.3 (14.7)	66	69.6 (16.9)		.0005
Socialization SS mean (SD)	96.7 (15.4)	66	70.8 (15.6)		.0005
Communication SS mean (SD)	99.3 (14.7)	66	77.4 (18.1)		.0005
Daily living skills SS mean (SD)	91.3 (13.5)	66	74.8 (20.4)		.0005
Full scale IQ mean (SD)	105.7 (16.2)	63	83.9 (20.5)		.0005
Performance IQ mean (SD)	105.0 (19.2)	63	84.7 (27.2)		.002
Verbal IQ mean (SD)	105.1 (13.7)	64	86.1 (16.0)		.0005
Psychosocial variables					
CRS global family function mean (SD)[c]	4.51 (1.3)	63	3.15 (1.1)	13	.001
Lifetime preinjury psychiatric disorder n (%)	21 (31)		4 (29)	12	ns
Family inventory of life events mean (SD)[d,e]	325.4 (250.3)	57	489.8 (313.3)		ns
Family psychiatric history mean (SD)	1.40 (1.1)	63	1.86 (1.0)		ns
Family history of ADHD (1st-degree relatives) n (%)	8 (13)	63	1 (7)		ns
Socioeconomic status mean (SD)	2.58 (1.1)		3.14 (1.0)		ns

Note. [a]n = 67 unless noted otherwise. [b]n = 14 unless noted otherwise. [c]The higher the CRS score, the more functional the family. CRS scores between 5 and 7 indicate healthy to superior family functioning, whereas scores between 1 and 4 indicate families in the clinical range (in need of family therapy). CRS scores between 5 and 7 (530–635) in a normal cohort on which the family inventory of life events was originally validated vary slightly with developmental stage of the family (e.g., [d]Mean scores those with preschool children vs. school-age children vs. adolescents). Scores above 735 to 950 are considered high. [e]Mann–Whitney U Test. TBI = traumatic brain injury; SADHD = secondary attention deficit hyperactivity disorder; SS = standard score; CRS = Clinical Rating Scale.

171

TABLE 6
Adaptive Behavior, Intellectual Function, and Psychosocial Adversity Variables in Severe TBI Participants With and Without SADHD

	No SADHD[a]	n	SADHD[b]	n	Significance (p)	Effect Size (d)
Timing of data collection in years postinjury (SD)	2.2 (.8)		2.3 (.8)		ns	.12
Adaptive behavior composite SS mean (SD)	88.2 (19.1)		65.8 (17.7)		.003	1.22
Socialization SS mean (SD)	89.7 (18.1)		68.2 (16.0)		.003	1.26
Communication SS mean (SD)	92.6 (18.8)		71.1 (17.0)		.004	1.20
Daily living skills SS mean (SD)	89.9 (19.3)		72.3 (23.5)		.03	0.82
Full scale IQ mean (SD)	97.7 (18.5)	22	78.5 (21.6)	22	.015	0.95
Performance IQ mean (SD)	96.4 (22.3)	22	77.0 (26.8)	22	.04	0.79
Verbal IQ mean (SD)	98.7 (14.0)	23	83.3 (17.3)	23	.011	0.98
Psychosocial variables						
CRS global family function mean (SD)	4.04 (1.4)	23	3.22 (1.1)	9	ns	.65
Lifetime preinjury psychiatric disorder n (%)	8 (33)		1 (10)		ns	
Family inventory of life events[c] mean (SD)	306.1 (251.6)	21	478.5 (307.3)	8	ns	.61
Family psychiatric history in 1st-degree relatives (SD)	1.26 (1.1)	23	2.00 (0.9)		ns	.73
Family history of ADHD (1st-degree relatives) n (%)	2 (9)	23	1 (10)		ns	
Socioeconomic status mean (SD)	2.8 (1.0)		3.3 (1.1)		ns	.48

Note. TBI = traumatic brain injury; SADHD = secondary attention deficit hyperactivity disorder; SS = standard score; CRS = Clinical Rating Scale.
[a]n = 24. [b]n = 10. [c]Mann–Whitney U test.

psychosocial variables was significantly worse in the SADHD group, although effect sizes were in the "medium" range (Cohen, 1988; Table 6).

DISCUSSION

The study demonstrated for the first time that SADHD is clearly associated with increasing severity of injury. This was particularly evident when participants with a broad range of severity (mild, moderate, and severe TBI) were included in the analyses. These data are consistent with previous findings that new symptoms of ADHD after TBI were associated with increasing severity of TBI (Knights et al., 1991; Max, Arndt, et al., 1998). Interestingly, when only severe TBI children remained in the analyses, severity of injury no longer differentiated the groups with and without SADHD. The latter finding is consistent with another study that also had a restricted range of severity (Gerring et al., 1998) and is in contrast to Personality Change due to TBI, which is associated with severity of injury even within a restricted range of severity (Max et al., 2000). This may suggest that, although these disorders are related to each other and both clearly have significant injury–dose–response relations, SADHD outcome may be relatively more influenced by noninjury, for example, psychosocial, factors.

Due to the frequency of TBI in childhood and the known impact of ADHD on psychosocial functioning, improving the prediction of outcome regarding SADHD in individual children who have sustained a TBI is critical from scientific, clinical, and legal points of view. These data illustrate that almost one third of children with severe TBI develop SADHD. It appears that the severe nature of the injury is capable of causing SADHD independent of whether the child had symptoms of ADHD before the injury. Notably, SADHD is not necessarily a permanent complication and resolved in almost one third within 18 months postinjury. We found that one moderate TBI participant developed SADHD, but that this occurred only in the presence of preinjury traits of ADHD. A larger sample of participants with moderate TBI is needed to determine whether ADHD develops in this severity class only in the presence of preinjury traits. It would be ideal to elucidate whether the change from traits to the full ADHD syndrome was related to brain injury or to natural history. This would require inclusion of a group of non-TBI children with traits of ADHD controlling for age, gender, and SES, or an epidemiological study following a large cohort of children and observing the natural history of both TBI and ADHD. We found that SADHD occurs at a similar rate after mild–moderate TBI and orthopedic injury. Furthermore, the development of SADHD (and worsening of preinjury ADHD) in orthopedic injury participants is instructive in that changes in ADHD symptomatology need not necessarily be related to brain injury per se.

SADHD was associated with significant impairment in intellectual and adaptive function both when participants with a broad range of injury severity were included and when only participants with severe injury were analyzed. This finding is not surprising in a full range of severity classification, and is naturally related to the fact that SADHD was associated with significantly greater injury severity. Numerous studies have linked intellectual and adaptive function deficits with severity of TBI in children (Fay et al., 1994). However, the similar finding in the severe TBI-only analyses suggests that SADHD is clinically significant not only because of its behavioral complications but also because of associated functional impairments in other domains including cognitive and adaptive function. These findings were robust despite the design weakness that two versions of the WISC were used and the use of digit span in the derivation of VIQ in Study 2.

SADHD was associated with significantly greater family dysfunction when participants with mild-to-severe TBI were considered but not when only severe TBI children were included. "Medium" effect sizes suggest that this may be related to lack of power in the latter analysis. Our finding that measures of family life events were neither elevated nor significantly different between SADHD and non-SADHD groups were in contrast to a previous study that used an instrument designed to measure family burden specific to TBI (Armstrong et al., 2001). In addition to the dose–response relation of TBI and SADHD, the negative finding regarding familial ADHD and SADHD may be further indication that traumatic neuronal damage is implicated in the manifestation of SADHD.

Analyses of lesion location failed to distinguish between severe TBI participants with and without SADHD. This may be related to the quality of the imaging data. CT scans are sensitive in the detection of lesions relevant to neurosurgical decision making after TBI, but are relatively insensitive in detection of diffuse injuries, subcortical lesions, and small lesions. If SADHD were linked with diffuse axonal injury (as suggested by the duration of impaired consciousness and GCS data rather than the lesion location and lesion area), then no lesion–behavior correlate would be anticipated. Perhaps magnetic resonance imaging would be more likely to demonstrate a subcortical lesion-specific correlation with SADHD (Gerring et al., 2000; Herskovits et al., 1999).

CONCLUSION

SADHD is associated with increasing severity of childhood TBI and is an important psychiatric syndrome associated with decrements in intellectual, adaptive, and family functioning. There is little doubt that SADHD can be induced by severe TBI. However, it is unclear whether it occurs after moderate TBI in the absence of preinjury ADHD symptoms. Conclusive proof that SADHD is related to the direct effects of brain injury characteristic of mild TBI is lacking. Extensive work is necessary to clarify injury, genetic, and psychosocial risk factors as well as the pathophysiology of SADHD.

ACKNOWLEDGMENT

This research was supported by a National Alliance for Research in Schizophrenia and Affective Disorders Young Investigator Award and an National Institute of Mental Health K 08 MH01800 Award (to Jeffrey E. Max).

REFERENCES

American Psychiatric Association. (1987). *Diagnostic and statistical manual of mental disorders* (3rd ed., rev.). Washington, DC: Author.

Andreasen, N. C., Endicott, J., Spitzer, R. L., & Winokur, G. (1977). The family history method using research diagnostic criteria: Reliability and validity. *Archives of General Psychiatry, 34,* 1229–1235.

Armstrong, K., Janusz, J., Yeates, K. O., Taylor, H. G., Wade, S., Stancin, T., et al. (2001). Long-term attention problems in children with traumatic brain injuries. *Journal of the International Neuropsychological Association, 7,* 238.

Biederman, J., Faraone, S. V., Doyle, A., Lehman, B. K., Kraus, I., Perrin, J., et al. (1993). Convergence of the child behavior checklist with structured interview-based psychiatric diagnoses of ADHD children with and without comorbidity. *Jounal of Child Psychology and Psychiatry, 34,* 1241–1251.

Bloom, D. R., Levin, H. S., Ewing-Cobbs, L., Saunders, A. E. Song, J., Fletcher, J. M., & et al. (2001). Lifetime and novel psychiatric disorders after pediatric traumatic brain injury. *Journal of the American Academy of Child and Adolescent Psychiatry, 40,* 572–579.

Brown, G., Chadwick, O., Shaffer, D., Rutter, M., & Traub, M. (1981). A prospective study of children with head injuries: III. Psychiatric Sequelae. *Psychological Medicine, 11,* 63–78.

Chambers, W. J., Puig-Antich, J., Hirsch, M., Paez, P., Ambrosini, P. J., Tabrizi, M. A., et al. (1985). The assessment of affective disorders in children and adolescents by semistructured interview: Test-retest reliability of the schedule for affective disorders and schizophrenia for school-age children, present episode version. *Archives of General Psychiatry, 42,* 696–702.

Cohen, J. (1988). *Statistical power analysis for the behavioral sciences.* Hillsdale, NJ: Lawrence Erlbaum Associates, Inc.

Damasio, H., & Damasio, A. R. (1989). *Lesion analysis in neuropsychology.* New York: Oxford University Press.

Faraone, S. V., Biederman, J., & Milberger, S. (1995). How reliable are maternal reports of their children's psychopathology? One-year recall of psychiatric diagnoses of ADHD children. *Journal of the American Academy of Child and Adolescent Psychiatry, 34,* 1001–1008.

Fay, G. C., Jaffe, K. M., Polissar, N. L., Liao, S., Rivara, J. B., & Martin, K. M. (1994). Outcome of pediatric traumatic brain injury at three years: A cohort study. *Archives of Physical Medicine and Rehabilitation, 75,* 733–741.

Gerring, J., Brady, K., Chen, A., Quinn, C., Herskovits, E., Bandeen-Roche, K., et al. (2000). Neuroimaging variables related to development of secondary attention deficit hyperactivity disorder after closed head injury in children and adolescents. *Brain Injury, 14,* 205–218.

Gerring, J. P., Brady, K. D., Chen, A., Vasa, R., Grados, M., Bandeen-Roche, K. J., et al. (1998). Premorbid prevalence of ADHD and development of secondary ADHD after closed head injury. *Journal of the American Academy of Child and Adolescent Psychiatry, 37,* 647–654.

Herskovits, E. H., Megalooikonomou, V., Davatzikos, C., Chen, A., Bryan, R. N., & Gerring, J. P. (1999). Is the spatial distribution of brain lesions associated with closed-head injury predictive of subsequent development of attention-deficit/hyperactivity disorder? Analysis with brain-image database. *Radiology, 213,* 389–394.

Hollingshead, A. B. (1975). *Four factor index of social status.* New Haven, CT: Yale University, Department of Sociology.

Kaufman, A. S., Ishikuma, T., & Kaufman-Packer, J. L. (1991). Amazingly short forms of the WAIS-R. *Journal of Psychoeducational Assessment, 9,* 4–15.

Kraus, J. F., Fife, D., & Conroy, C. (1987). Pediatric brain injuries: The nature, clinical course, and early outcomes in a defined United States' population. *Pediatrics, 79,* 501–507.

Knights, R. M., Ivan, L. P., Ventureyra, E. C. G., Bentivoglio, C., Stoddart, C., Winogron, W., et al. (1991), The effects of head injury in children on neuropsychological and behavioral functioning. *Brain Injury, 5,* 339–351.

Max, J. E., Arndt, S., Castillo, C. S., Bokura, H., Robin, D. A., Lindgren, S. D., et al. (1998). Attention deficit hyperactivity symptomatology after traumatic brain injury: A prospective study. *Journal of the American Academy of Child Adolescent Psychiatry, 37,* 841–847.

Max, J. E., Castillo, C. S., Lindgren, S. D., & Arndt, S. V. (1998). The Neuropsychiatric Rating Schedule: Reliability and validity. *Journal of the American Academy of Child and Adolescent Psychiatry, 37,* 297–304.

Max, J. E., Koele, S. L., Castillo, C. S., Lindgren, S. D., Arndt, S., Bokura, H., et al. (2000). Personality change disorder in children and adolescents following traumatic brain injury. *Journal of the International Neuropsychological Society, 6,* 279–285.

Max, J. E., Koele, S. L., Smith, W. L., Sato, Y., Lindgren, S. D., Robin, D. A., et al. (1998). Psychiatric disorders in children and adolescents after severe traumatic brain injury: A controlled study. *Journal of the American Academy of Child and Adolescent Psychiatry, 37,* 832–840.

Max, J. E., Lindgren, S. D., Knutson, C., Pearson, S., Ihrig, D., & Welborn, A. (1997). Child and adolescent traumatic brain injury: psychiatric findings from a paediatric outpatient speciality clinic. *Brain Injury, 11,* 699–711.

Max, J. E., Lindgren, S. D., Knutson, C., Pearson, C. S., Ihrig, D., & Welborn, A. (1998). Child and adolescent traumatic brain injury: correlates of disruptive behavior disorders. *Brain Injury, 12,* 41–52.

Max, J. E., Robin, D. A., Lindgren, S. D., Smith, W. L., Sato, Y., Mattheis, P. J., et al. (1997). Traumatic brain injury in children and adolescents: Psychiatric disorders at two years. *Journal of the American Academy of Child and Adolescent Psychiatry, 36,* 1278–1285.

Max, J. E., Smith, W. L., Sato, Y., Mattheis, P. J., Castillo, C. S., Lindgren, S. D., et al. (1997). Traumatic brain injury in children and adolescents: psychiatric disorders in the first three months. *Journal of the American Academy of Child and Adolescent Psychiatry, 36,* 94–102.

McCubbin, H. I., Patterson, J. M., & Wilson, L. (1980). Family inventory of life events and changes (FILE) form A. In H. I. McCubbin & A. Thompson (Eds.), *Family assessment for research and practice* (pp. 97–98). Madison, WI: University of Wisconsin.

Miller, I. W., Kabacoff, R. I., Epstein, N. B., Bishop, D. S., Keitner, G. I., Baldwin, L. M., et al. (1994). The development of a clinical rating scale for the McMaster model of family functioning. *Family Process, 33,* 53–69.

Orvaschel, H., Puig-Antich, J., Chamber, W., Tabrizi, M. A., & Johnson, R. (1982). Retrospective assessment of prepubertal major depression with the Kiddie-SADS-E. *Journal of the American Academy of Child Psychiatry, 21,* 392–397.

Pless, I. B., Taylor, H. G., & Arsenault, L. (1995). The relationship between vigilance deficits and traffic injuries involving children. *Pediatrics, 95,* 219–224.

Sparrow, S. S., Balla, D., & Cicchetti, D. (1984). *The Vineland Adaptive Behavior Scales.* Circle Pines, MN: American Guidance Services.

Szatmari, P., Offord, D. R., & Boyle, M. H. (1989). Ontario child health study: prevalence of attention deficit disorder with hyperactivity. *Journal of Child Psychology and Psychiatry, 30,* 219–230.

Teasdale, G., & Jennett, B. (1974). Assessment of coma and impaired consciousness: A practical scale. *Lancet, 2,* 81–84.

Wechsler, D. (1974). *Wechsler Intelligence Scale for Children-Revised manual.* New York: The Psychological Corporation.

Wechsler, D. (1991). *Wechsler Intelligence Scale for Children-Third Edition.* New York: Psychological Corporation.

Williams, D. H., Levin, H. S., & Eisenberg, H. M. (1990). Mild head injury classification. *Neurosurgery, 27,* 422–428.

DEVELOPMENTAL NEUROPSYCHOLOGY, 25(1&2), 179–198
Copyright © 2004, Lawrence Erlbaum Associates, Inc.

Attention Deficit Hyperactivity Disorder Symptoms and Response Inhibition After Closed Head Injury in Children: Do Preinjury Behavior and Injury Severity Predict Outcome?

Russell Schachar
Brain and Behavior Program, Research Institute
Hospital for Sick Children
Toronto, Ontario, Canada

Harvey S. Levin
Cognitive Neuroscience Laboratory
Departments of Physical Medicine and Rehabilitation, Neurosurgery, and
Psychiatry and Behavioral Sciences
Baylor College of Medicine
Houston, TX

Jeffrey E. Max
Department of Psychiatry
University of California, San Diego
Children's Hospital and Health Center, San Diego

Karen Purvis
Department of Psychiatry
University of Iowa

Requests for reprints should be sent to Russell Schachar, Brain and Behavior Program, Research Institute, Hospital for Sick Children, 555 University Avenue, Toronto, Ontario, Canada M5G 1X8. E-mail: russell.schachar@sickkids.ca

Shirley Chen
Department of Psychiatry
Hospital for Sick Children
Toronto, Ontario, Canada

We examined the effect of closed head injury (CHI) on the development of symptoms of secondary attention deficit hyperactivity disorder (SADHD), emotional disturbance, and impaired response inhibition. We also investigated the relation of developmental and recovery variables to SADHD symptoms and inhibition. Participants were 200 children aged 5–17 years, 137 children who had CHI, and 63 children with no history of CHI served as controls. We assessed preinjury behavior problems, head injury variables (severity, age at time of injury, time since injury), postinjury SADHD, and anxiety symptoms at least 2 years following the head injury. Response inhibition was measured with the stop-signal task. CHI predicted the development of SADHD symptoms and anxiety with more severe injury predicting more severe outcomes. Only the combination of severe CHI and a high level of SADHD symptoms predicted poor response inhibition. Postinjury anxiety was not associated with poor inhibition. The consequences of CHI did not vary with age at injury or time since injury, but poorer outcome was predicted by preinjury behavior problems. CHI in children leads to SADHD symptoms and anxiety even after taking preinjury disturbance into account. Poor response inhibition is a consequence of CHI but only when the CHI is severe and the child manifests high levels of SADHD symptoms.

Closed head injury (CHI) in childhood results in a wide range of behavioral, cognitive, and emotional consequences (Dennis, Guger, Roncadin, Barnes, & Schachar, 2001). Among the behavioral problems that follow CHI, inattentiveness, restlessness and impulsiveness are particularly common. These symptoms are prominent, as well, in primary or developmental attention deficit hyperactivity disorder (ADHD). Hereditary neurophysiological or neurochemical abnormality rather than acquired brain injury appears to make the largest contribution to the development of ADHD (Eaves et al., 1997; Thapar, Holmes, Poulton, & Harrington, 1999). As a result of the similarity in behavioral manifestations, the syndrome of inattention, restlessness, and impulsiveness arising after CHI is known as secondary ADHD (SADHD). SADHD develops in approximately 20% of previously unaffected individuals (Gerring et al., 1998; Max, Koele, et al., 1998; Max, Lindgren, et al., 1998; Max, Robin, et al., 1998). The high probability of developing SADHD following CHI suggests that it may be a consequence of brain injury to the frontal lobes. This hypothesis is compatible with the high frequency of frontal-lobe contusions after CHI and the proposed role of frontal regions in self-regulation and behavioral control (Di Stefano et al., 2000; Herskovits et al., 1999; Levin et al., 1993; Levin & Kraus 1994; Levin et al., 2000; Mendelsohn et al., 1992; Miller & Cohen 2001).

However, children with ADHD and individuals who are restless, inattentive, and impulsive tend to be accident-prone risk takers (Barkley 1997; Barkley, Guevremont, Anastopoulos, DuPaul, & Shelton 1993; Barkley, Murphy, & Kwasnik, 1996; Bijur, Golding, Haslum, & Kurzon, 1988). Consequently, they may be overrepresented in samples of children with CHI (Gerring et al., 1998). If so, premorbid ADHD symptoms rather than brain trauma per se may account for some portion of the increased risk of postinjury SADHD. The first specific aim of this study, therefore, was to explore the link between CHI and SADHD symptoms following CHI. If there is a causal relation between CHI and SADHD, then SADHD should develop following CHI in children without preinjury ADHD, and CHI should predict SADHD symptom severity beyond that which is attributable to preinjury behavior. Evidence for a causal relation of CHI and SADHD would be strengthened if variation in CHI severity accounted for variation in severity of SADHD manifestations. The relation of CHI and SADHD could also be a function of the emotional impact of the injury rather than brain injury per se. If brain injury rather than emotional factors underlie the increase in SADHD after CHI, CHI variables should account for more of the variation in SADHD symptoms than in anxiety symptoms.

In addition to behavioral dysfunction, CHI results in various cognitive impairments. For example, CHI results in deficits in sustained, focused, and selective attention and in response execution (Dennis, Wilkinson, Koski, & Humphreys, 1995; Ewing-Cobbs et al., 1998; Kaufmann, Fletcher, Levin, Miner, & Ewing-Cobbs, 1993; Levin et al., 1993; Levin et al., 1988; Murray, Shum, & McFarland, 1992; Robin, Max, Steirwalt, Guenzer, & Lindgren, 1999). In particular, CHI results in impairment of inhibition of prepotent (Dennis et al., 1995; Konrad, Gauggel, Manz, & Scholl, 2000) and ongoing responses (Konrad et al., 2000). Similar deficits in inhibition have been identified consistently in ADHD (Daugherty, Quay, & Ramos, 1993; Schachar & Logan 1990; Schachar, Mota, Logan, Tannock, & Klim, 2000; Schachar & Tannock, 1995; Schachar, Tannock, & Logan, 1993; Solanto, 1990; Solanto, Abikoff, Sonuga-Barke, Schachar, Logan, Wigal, et al., 2001; cf. Kuntsi, Oosterlaan, & Stevenson, 2001). Indeed, inhibitory deficit is regarded as the central deficit in ADHD according to several current theories (Barkley 1997; Quay, 1988, 1997). Therefore, it is somewhat unexpected that neither Dennis et al. (2001) nor Konrad et al. (2000) observed a correlation between the extent of the inhibition deficit and the severity of SADHD manifestations in children with CHI. These findings question the link between inhibition deficit and ADHD behavior. Consequently, the second aim of this study was to examine the relation of SADHD symptoms and the putative cognitive marker of ADHD, inhibition deficit.

The third aim of this study was to investigate the relation of developmental variables to SADHD and response inhibition. Regardless of injury severity, children with a younger age at the time of CHI generally have poorer cognitive performance compared to those with a later age at injury (Dennis et al., 2001, for review). Cognitive deficits persist from the acute stage (Chadwick, 1985; Chadwick, Rutter, Brown, Shaffer, & Traub, 1981; Chadwick, Rutter, Shaffer, & Shrout, 1981) into the chronic stage of CHI with no clear improvement (Catroppa, Anderson, & Stargatt, 1999; Dennis et al., 1995; Kaufmann et al., 1993). Moreover, cognitive impairment worsens with increasing severity of CHI (Dennis et al., 2001). The association of CHI severity, age at the time of injury, time since injury and response inhibition has not been studied extensively (cf. Konrad et al., 2000). It is not clear if the behavioral consequences of CHI are more severe in children who were injured at a younger age (Dennis et al., 2001, for review) or if behavior improves with the passage of time. To investigate these issues, we explored the association between age at the time of CHI, time since the injury, SADHD symptoms, and response inhibition after CHI.

METHOD

Research Participants

Participants were 200 children aged 5–17 years, 137 children who had CHI, and 63 children with no history of CHI served as controls. CHI participants were assessed and treated in one of several large, urban pediatric hospitals in Toronto, Dallas, or Houston at least 2 years prior to the study. Controls were recruited by advertisement in local newspapers. CHI and control cases were assessed in the same way.

Participants were excluded if they had a history of ADHD, learning disability, or speech–language delay antedating the head injury. Exclusion and inclusion criteria were established by parent interview and were based on history that the child had been diagnosed or treated for the condition, for example, placement in a special class for children with learning problems or treatment with psychostimulant medication. Interviewers were PhD level clinical psychologists or child psychiatrists.

Behavioral Measures

Preinjury disturbance.   Based on parental description of child behavior prior to the head injury, interviewers coded the presence of short attention span, underachievement, and overactivity. This history was obtained retrospectively at the time of assessment, which was at least 2 years after the CHI. Preinjury behavioral disturbance was coded in the controls based on behavior during preschool years.

Postinjury disturbance.   The Survey Diagnostic Instrument (SDI) served as the primary measure of postinjury SADHD and anxiety. The SDI allows for rating of all symptoms required to make major DSM diagnoses with reliability and predictive validity that equals structured interviews (Boyle et al., 1997). Parents *and* teachers completed SDI questionnaires for each participant based on behavior during the past 6 months. We derived quantitative and categorical measures of SADHD and anxiety from these scores. The *sum* of parent and teacher ratings of ADHD and of anxiety symptoms provided an index of overall behavioral disturbance. A research diagnosis of SADHD was assigned if parent *or* teacher scores exceeded the threshold (mean plus 1 *SD*) for ADHD using age and gender norms that were derived from general population of children (Boyle et al., 1996). A research diagnosis of anxiety was assigned in a similar way.

Head injury severity. Information for the Glasgow Coma Scale (GCS; Teasdale & Jennett, 1974) was abstracted from the medical record of participants in the absence of any knowledge of the child's course and outcome. GCS is based on movement, eye opening, and verbal responsiveness. GCS ratings were taken as the lowest, postresuscitation assigned GCS score in the ambulance or on admission to the emergency room. A quantitative GCS score varied from 3 (unresponsive) to 15 (normal). Children were divided into three head injury severity categories— mild (GCS = 13–15), moderate (GCS = 9–12), or severe (GCS = 3–8).

Inhibitory control. We measured response inhibition with the stop-signal task. The stop-signal task is a laboratory analogue of a situation that requires rapid and accurate execution of a simple motor action and, occasional and unpredictable, cessation of this action (Logan, 1994). The paradigm involves two concurrent tasks, a *go task* and a *stop task*. The go task involves a choice among stimulus and response alternatives (discrimination of an *X* from an *O*). The object of the go task is to respond as quickly and accurately as possible. The stop signal occurs unpredictably on 25% of go-task trials and involves presentation of a signal (a tone) that instructs participants to completely stop their response to the go task on that trial. Whether or not children are able to inhibit on a particular trial depends on the outcome of a race between go (activation) and stop (inhibition) processes. If the stop-task response finishes before the go-task response, children will inhibit their response to the go task (Jennings, van der Molen, Brock, & Somsen, 1992; Jennings, van der Molen, Pelham, Debski, & Hoza, 1997; Logan, 1985, 1994; Logan, Cowan, & Davis, 1984; Olman, 1973; Osman, Kornblum, & Meyer, 1986). If the go-task response finishes before the stop-task response, children will fail to inhibit their response to the go task, responding much as they would if no stop signal had been presented. Thus, inhibitory control depends on the latency of two independent processes—the response to the go signal (go reaction time, GoRT) and the response to the stop signal (stop-signal reaction time, SSRT). The outcome of the race between the go and stop processes depends as well on the interval between the onset of the go signal and the onset of the stop signal (stop-signal delay). Short delay between the go and stop signals increases the probability of inhibiting and long delay increases the probability of responding.

We employed a new method of calculating SSRT (Logan, 1994; Logan, Schachar, & Tannock, 1997). This method uses a tracking algorithm to find a stop-signal delay that ties the race between the go process and the stop process. The algorithm increases stop-signal delay when children inhibit successfully, and it decreases stop-signal delay when children fail to inhibit. If the increments and decrements are equal in magnitude (50-msec changes), the algorithm will converge on a stop-signal delay at which children inhibit 50% of the time. At that point, the go process and the stop process finish at the same time, on average. Go-signal reaction time and stop-signal delay are observable. SSRT is unobservable but can be estimated simply by subtracting stop-signal delay from mean go-signal reaction time (Logan et al., 1997). Calculated in this way, SSRT is a precise measure of latency of an internally generated, although unobserved, inhibitory control process independent of go-signal reaction time. Compared to individuals with good inhibitory control, those with poor inhibitory control will have longer SSRT. The tracking algorithm also takes into account the nature of the strategy that a person adopts to perform the go task. Individuals who respond quickly to the go task will have shorter stop-signal delay; individuals with slower go responses or who "wait" for the stop signal will have longer stop-signal delays. In either case, the outcome of the race will be biased in the same way and SSRT can be calculated if, on average, individuals inhibit on 50% of trials.

The stimuli for the go task were the upper-case letters X and O (1.25 in. in height), presented in the center of the screen for 1,000 msec. Each trial is preceded by a 500-msec fixation point, presented in the center of the screen and then extinguished. The screen remains blank for 2000 msec. Consequently, each trial includes a period of 3.5 sec in which the child can respond to the primary task in accordance with the task's demands. The stop signal is a tone of 1,000 Hz. Responses is recorded with hand-held response box with buttons labeled with either an X or an O. Identical response buttons were used at each site.

The stop task was presented in a game-like fashion in eight blocks. Each block consisted of 32 trials—24 go signal trials without stop signals and 8 trials that included a stop signal. The X and O stimuli, which comprised the go signals, occurred equally often in each block. Children were instructed to keep the index finger of their left hand on the X button and the index finger of their right hand on the O button throughout the experiment. Children were encouraged to continue responding to the go signal as quickly and as accurately as possible if no stop signal was presented. They were told that stop signals occur in such a way that sometimes it would be difficult to stop and sometimes not. Stop-signal delay was set initially at 250 msec. Participant's performance was monitored throughout the task and they were reminded about the importance of maintaining the speed and accuracy of their responses to the go signal. Go reaction time (GoRT), percent inhibition (PSR), and SSRT were calculated for each experimental block.

Accuracy, percentage of inhibition, and SSRT were examined to determine whether the individual had generally complied with the requirements of the task. Acceptable performance was defined as fewer than 33% invalid trials (no responses on go task) and more than 66% correct responses to the go task (indicating that the participant was engaged in the primary task). Based on the modeling of Band (1997), we also excluded participants who obtained SSRT less than 50 msec, Go RT less than 100 msec or greater than 2,000 msec, or PSR less than 12.5 or more than 87.5.

Analysis

We compared head injury severity groups and controls on categorical variables with chi-square and on continuous variables with analysis of variance (ANOVA). The effects of head injury severity and SADHD on response inhibition were analyzed using ANOVA with two levels of SADHD (present, absent) and three levels of head injury severity (mild, moderate, and severe). The same approach was used to examine the effects of postinjury anxiety and CHI on response inhibition.

Linear regression analyses were used to assess the relation between head injury severity (GCS) and postinjury behavior scores (SADHD, anxiety) after controlling premorbid behavioral problem, age at injury, age at time of assessment, time since injury, and gender. Multiple linear regression was performed using GCS on CHI participants only because no GCS score exists for controls. A linear regression model was run on all participants using the 4-point scale of head injury severity (*mild, moderate, severe,* and *no CHI,* i.e., controls) to see the relation between head injury and behavior scores. Regression analyses were also use to see if head injury affects stop-signal task performance after controlling age and gender. The analyses began with a saturated model and proceeded with backward elimination of nonsignificant terms. The goodness of fit of the resulting model was evaluated with the R-squared coefficient (R^2).

RESULTS

Participant Characteristics

Five CHI subjects had no GCS recorded. Thirteen of the 132 CHI participants (9.8%) had a confirmed diagnosis of ADHD (4), learning disability, (5) and/or speech–language delay (5) prior to head injury, whereas six of the 63 controls had one of these diagnoses (9.5%). These children were excluded from further analyses.

Demographic characteristics of CHI groups and controls are presented in Table 1. Age at time of injury varied from 0.4 to 13.7 years. The severe CHI group was older than the mild CHI group at the time of injury ($t = 2.4, p < .05$). CHI children were significantly older than control children at the time of the assessment ($t = -2.1, p < .05$) but no significant difference was observed among the CHI severity groups. Time since the injury varied from 2.1 to 15 years but did not differ among the CHI groups ($F = 0.9, ns$). The means of GCS were 5.4 ($SD = 1.8$), 10.4 ($SD = 1.2$), and 14.6 ($SD = 0.6$), respectively, for severe, moderate, and mild head injury group.

Behavioral Disturbance

Behavioral problems such as short attention span, underachievement, or overactivity prior to head injury were reported in 41.5% ($N = 61$) of children with CHI. Of these 61 children, 12.9% ($n = 19$) children had one problem, 21.1% ($n = 31$) had two problems, and 7.5% ($n = 11$) had three problems. The most common behavioral problem was short attention span (91.8% of reported problems, $n = 56$). The CHI children (49.5%) had a greater proportion of behavior problem prior to head injury than the control children (25%) during preschool ($\chi^2 = 7.89, p < .01$) but the three CHI severity groups did not differ in the rate of behavioral problems prior to their CHI ($\chi^2 = 0.18, ns$).

CHI children (35.6%) were significantly more likely than controls (11.8%) to meet criteria for a research diagnosis of SADHD at the time of assessment ($\chi^2 = 6.8, p < .01$). However, the various head injury severity groups did not differ in prevalence of postinjury SADHD ($\chi^2 = 0.26, ns$; see also quantitative scores, Table 1). The prevalence of postinjury anxiety symptoms, by comparison, did not differ between the CHI groups (23.8%) and the controls (17.6%, $\chi^2 = 0.53, ns$) and no significant difference in rate of anxiety was observed among three CHI severity groups ($\chi^2 = 3.7, ns$). However, analyses of quantitative anxiety scores indicated a dose–response relation whereby greater CHI severity was associated with greater postanxiety scores ($F = 5.22, p < .01$).

Regression analysis showed that postinjury SADHD scores were predicted by preinjury behavioral problems ($\beta = .66, p < .001$) and by GCS ($\beta = -0.18, p < .05$). More severe CHI and greater preinjury behavior problems predicted greater postinjury SADHD symptoms. Age at injury, age at time of assessment, time since injury, and sex were not related to postinjury SADHD scores.

Teacher and parent ratings of SADHD behaviors were significantly correlated ($.47, p < .001$). Parent SADHD ratings ($N = 105$) were predicted by preinjury behavior problems and GCS. Teacher SADHD ratings ($N = 80$) were predicted by preinjury behavior problems but not by GCS although the direction of the relation was similar to that observed for parent ratings.

TABLE 1
Demographic Characteristics of Groups

	Controls[a]	Mild CHI[b]	Moderate CHI[c]	Severe CHI[d]	F/χ^2	p
Age (years) at test ($M \pm SD$)	11.1 (3.1)	11.2 (3.5)	12.3 (2.8)	12.54 (2.7)	2.4	>.05
Age (years) at injury ($M \pm SD$)		6.1 (3.3)	6.9 (2.6)	7.65 (3.2)	2.9	.059
Time since CHI (years)		5.1(2.1)	5.0(2.1)	4.77 (1.4)	0.9	>.05
Sex (% male)	45.6	58.5	70.0	64.7	5.3	>.05
GCS		14.6 (0.6)	10.4(1.2)	5.4 (1.8)		
Preinjury behavioral problems (%)	25.0	50.0	52.9	46.7	8.2	<.05
Short attention span	20.4	45.5	52.9	40.0	9.4	<.05
Underachievement	12.2	28.8	41.2	26.7	7.2	>.05
Overactivity	12.2	20.4	35.3	16.7	4.6	>.05
Symptom scores						
SADHD	8.2 (10.1)	12.8 (11.6)	11.6 (11.1)	14.2 (9.3)	1.8	>.05
Anxiety	3.6 (2.6)	4.2 (2.9)	4.7 (2.9)	6.6 (3.9)	5.2	<.05
Research diagnosis						
SADHD(%)	11.8	33.3	37.5	38.5	7.0	>.05
Anxiety (%)	17.6	15.6	30.8	34.6	4.4	>.05

Note. CHI= closed head injury; GCS=Glasgow Coma Scale; SADHD = secondary attention deficit hyperactivity disorder.
[a]$n = 57$. [b]$n = 65$. [c]$n = 20$. [d]$n = 34$.

Because more severely injured children were older at the time of their injury, we repeated the regression analyses after excluding children younger than 2.4 years of age at the time of injury. Excluding younger children at the time of injury eliminated differences in age at injury among the severity groups. The results of the regression analysis remained the same: Age at injury did not predict the extent of SADHD symptoms following injury.

GCS scores ($\beta = -.38, p < .01$) but not other variables predicted postinjury anxiety scores. More severe CHI was associated with greater anxiety.

Stop-Signal Task Performance

Twenty participants were excluded because their scores did not meet criteria for acceptable performance on the stop-signal task. Children with and without valid stop-signal task data did not differ in age, SADHD or anxiety scores, gender, or preinjury behavior problems. However, a greater proportion of the severe CHI group compared to the mild or moderate groups were excluded because they had invalid stop-task data ($\chi^2 = 7.01, p < .05$).

Table 2 shows stop-signal task scores for participants with and without a research diagnosis of SADHD within each head injury severity group. ANOVA showed there are no effects of CHI severity group ($F = 1.06, p > 0.05$) and SADHD ($F = 0.017, p > 0.05$) for SSRT but the interaction between CHI severity group and SADHD was significant for SSRT, $F(2, 65) = 3.8, p < .05$. This interaction is attributed to the longer SSRT of those children with severe CHI and postinjury SADHD. Neither SADHD in the absence of severe head injury nor mild or moderate CHI conferred a risk for deficient inhibition. No main effects of CHI severity, SADHD, or the interaction between CHI severity and SADHD were found for mean go RT, percent correct, and percent inhibition.

As a result of the interaction between postinjury SADHD and CHI severity, we included the interaction between these two predictors in the regression model. Regression analysis identified preinjury behavioral problems, SADHD, the interaction between SADHD and CHI severity, age, and gender as significant predictors of SSRT. Younger children at the time of assessment ($\beta = -.32, p < .01$), children with SADHD ($\beta = -.83, p < .01$), those with greater preinjury behavioral problems ($\beta = .52, p < .001$), and females ($\beta = .33, p < .01$) had longer SSRT indicating poorer inhibition. The interaction between postinjury ADHD and CHI severity also predicted SSRT ($\beta = -.9, p < .001$). The interaction between SADHD and CHI severity indicated that, among SADHD children, more severely injured children had longer SSRT. When we assessed regression models separately for SADHD and non-SADHD cases, the effect of CHI severity was evident only in children with SADHD. Age at injury and time since injury did not predict SSRT. Postinjury anxiety did not enter the model as a predictor of SSRT.

TABLE 2
Stop Signal Task Performance

	Controls[a]	Mild CHI-ADHD[b]	Mild CHI-ADHD[c]	Moderate CHI-ADHD[d]	Moderate CHI-ADHD[e]	Severe CHI-ADHD[f]	Severe CHI-ADHD[g]
SSRT	263.9 (112.9)	290.6 (151.1)	289.0 (145.0)	274.9 (124.1)	283.7 (113.5)	181.2 (95.2)	418.7 (238.2)
Go RT	551.9 (155.8)	571.5 (120.3)	623.9 (241.8)	628.5 (156.0)	568.0 (65.9)	513.5 (111.2)	533.9 (119.8)
Percentage correct	95.2 (5.0)	94.9 (4.9)	96.3 (3.3)	93.1 (7.3)	93.1 (4.8)	97.3 (2.5)	94.2 (5.1)
Percentage of inhibition	51.4 (3.2)	50.4 (7.7)	52.0 (6.0)	52.1 (2.8)	48.8 (3.2)	51.0 (3.0)	44.6 (16.8)

Note. CHI = closed head injury; ADHD = attention deficit hyperactivity disorder; SSRT = stop signal reaction time.
[a] $n = 29$. [b] $n = 24$. [c] $n = 15$. [d] $n = 7$. [e] $n = 5$. [f] $n = 9$. [g] $n = 8$.

ANOVA did not indicate an effect of postinjury anxiety, CHI severity, or the interaction of these variables for SSRT (scores not shown). However, ANOVA indicated an interaction between postinjury anxiety and CHI severity for go RT, $F(2, 60) = 3.2, p < .05$. Among those with mild CHI, anxious children were slower to execute the response to the go task. Among those with moderate and severe CHI, anxious children were faster. The final regression model for go RT confirmed the interaction of anxiety and CHI severity ($\beta = -1.83, p < .01$).

DISCUSSION

This study examined the association between CHI and SADHD symptoms and between CHI and response inhibition in a large sample of children in the chronic stage of CHI and in control children without head injury or SADHD. We focused on response inhibition because a deficit in this component of executive control is commonly observed in ADHD even though it is only one of the various cognitive processes that can be perturbed by CHI. We evaluated the contribution of preinjury behavior disturbance, head injury severity, age at the time of injury, age at the time of assessment, and time since the injury to SADHD symptoms and to response inhibition. We excluded CHI children with a confirmed preinjury diagnosis of ADHD, language, or learning disability because these children are more likely to suffer CHI and to develop SADHD symptoms independent of the effect of brain trauma. To determine whether SADHD and response inhibition deficits are specific consequences of head injury, we examined the predictors of a contrasting postinjury behavioral disturbance, anxiety, and a contrasting cognitive ability, the speed of response execution.

SADHD symptoms were a clear consequence of CHI in this sample. A research diagnosis of SADHD was three times more common in children with CHI than in controls even after excluding individuals with clear-cut preexisting disorder. We observed a research diagnosis of SADHD in 35% of CHI cases, a rate that is broadly in line with previous reports (Fletcher et al., 1996; Gerring et al., 1998; Max et al., 1998; Max et al., 2004/this issue). Some of this increased risk for SADHD symptoms following injury was attributable to preinjury behavior disturbance. Nevertheless, preinjury behavioral disturbance did not account completely for postinjury SADHD symptoms. In strong support of the causal role of head injury, we observed a dose–response relation of head injury severity and SADHD (Max, Arndt, et al., 1998). More severely injured children were at greater risk for SADHD. Although the mechanism of this relation cannot be determined in this study, it is likely to involve damage to frontal and functionally related subcortical brain regions. Frontal areas are involved in higher order cognitive function, inhibition, and behavioral self-regulation (Miller & Cohen 2001); these areas are commonly injured in childhood CHI (Levin et al., 1993; Levin & Kraus 1994). Frontal dysfunction is also implicated in the etiology of both developmental (Filipek et al., 1997; Semrud-Clikeman et al., 1994) and secondary ADHD (Herskovits et al., 1999). Structural and functional brain imaging techniques would permit clearer understanding of the relation between response inhibition and the neural substrates involved in SADHD.

Deficient inhibition was evident only among children with a severe CHI and with SADHD. Neither the presence of postinjury SADHD nor CHI individually predicted deficient response inhibition. A previous study of CHI and SADHD using the stop-signal task did not detect a threshold effect of CHI severity on inhibition because it did not include children with a range of head injury severity (Konrad et al., 2000). Younger age in this sample of children with CHI also predicted relatively poorer inhibition, suggesting that CHI children may follow a developmental course that parallels that observed among normal children (Schachar & Logan 1990; Williams, Ponesse, Schachar, Logan, & Tannock, 1999). Female sex predicted poorer inhibition among individuals with CHI. This study is the first time that sex has been a predictor of inhibition in normal or pathological samples (Williams et al., 1999).

Broadly, the results support the idea of a specific relation of CHI, SADHD, and deficient response inhibition. First, no association of postinjury anxiety and poor inhibition was observed. Second, increasing severity of CHI did not predict generalized slowing of all cognitive processes as measured by the speed of Go responses. In fact, children with anxiety and mild CHI tended to be significantly slower. However, go reaction time in the stop-signal task is an imperfect index of cognitive slowing because it may reflect a combination of strategy, attention processes, and response activation. Nevertheless, the absence of an effect of CHI on go reaction time reinforces the interpretation that there is a specific relation among CHI, SADHD, and deficient response inhibition rather than a generalized cognitive deficit arising from CHI.

This study did not replicate earlier research pointing to a relation of age at injury and measures of vigilance and response modulation, processes that involve withholding a response (Dennis et al., 2001). The difference between these two studies probably arises from the fact that response withholding and response withdrawal reflect different underlying processes. Dennis et al. (2001) operationalized inhibition as withholding of a response using the Gordon Delay Task (Gordon, 1983, 1988), whereas this study measured withdrawal of a response that is already being executed. Withholding and withdrawing of responses may involve distinct neural substrates (Rubia et al., 2001).

This study did not replicate earlier studies in which cognition was found to improve with longer elapsed time since the injury (Dennis et al., 2001). The difference between these studies might lie in the fact that this sample was assessed well into the chronic stage of their CHI and well beyond the period of active recovery.

The data bear on views about the association between primary or developmental ADHD and secondary or acquired ADHD. Deficient inhibition has been recorded in the majority of studies in primary ADHD (Oosterlaan, Logan, & Sergeant, 1998). Moreover, deficient inhibition has not been observed in other childhood psychopathologies such as conduct disorder or anxiety (Oosterlaan et al., 1998; Schachar et al., 2000). A recent study supported the possibility that deficient response inhibition among ADHD individuals may delineate a particularly heritable subtype of ADHD (Crosbie & Schachar, 2001). These data support the hypothesis that an inhibition deficit measured by the stop-signal task may be more strongly related to primary ADHD than to SADHD arising following CHI. This study indicates that acquired brain dysfunction can cause the same deficit as that observed in primary ADHD but only in severely injured children. Those with mild or moderate CHI did not show a deficit. And it is noteworthy that deficient inhibition was evident only in those with SADHD as well as severe CHI. Taken together, these data reinforce the importance of an inhibition deficit in ADHD and suggest that studies of lesions in SADHD with deficit in response inhibition might clarify the nature of the deficit in ADHD.

Compared with other samples of CHI children, there were relatively few individuals in this sample with ADHD prior to their head injury. We identified only 4 (3%) among the 137 CHI cases with a history of ADHD antedating their head injury. In previous CHI samples, 10% to 30% of cases were judged to have had preinjury ADHD (Gerring et al., 1998; Max et al., 2004/this issue; Konrad et al., 2000). The difference may lie in the younger age at injury of participants in this study (6–7.5 years) compared to other studies (e.g., 9.1 years; Konrad et al., 2000). The children in this study may have been too young to receive assessment or treatment despite marked behavioral disturbance. The difference may also be due to the method of assessment of preinjury behavioral disturbance and to the criteria used for defining preinjury ADHD. We based a research diagnosis of preinjury ADHD on a history of a diagnosis of ADHD made by a professional prior to CHI, or on the basis of treatment for ADHD with medication or special class placement. Other studies have based preinjury ADHD on parental report (Gerring et al., 1998; Konrad et al., 2000). It is likely that retrospective diagnostic methods would result in some degree of diagnostic error arising from variation in referral patterns and clinical practices in the community.

On the other hand, some support for our method of assessing preinjury behavior is evident in the fact that hyperactive, inattentive, and impulsive behavior presented a risk for CHI even after excluding cases with a research diagnosis of preinjury ADHD. Half of the CHI group but only 25% of controls were described as exhibiting short attention span, underachievement, or overactivity prior to their injury. Although these cases did not have an established ADHD diagnoses, it was evident that their problems were severe based on the fact that a number of individuals had more than one of these problems. It may be that some of these children would have been diagnosed with ADHD or learning disability with the passage of time even in the absence of a CHI. These findings are consistent with previous studies showing that children with ADHD symptoms are over represented in samples of children with CHI (Max et al., 1998). Furthermore, these results confirm earlier studies that relate restless, inattentive, and impulsive behavior to increased risk for engagement in dangerous behavior (Barkley et al., 1993; Bijur et al., 1988; Bijur, Stewart-Brown, & Butler, 1986) and, subsequently, head injury. Finally, this observation supports the hypothesis that preinjury subclinical problems can develop into full disorders after head injury (Asarnow, Satz, Light, Lewis, & Neumann, 1991; Brown, Chadwick, Shaffer, Rutter, & Traub, 1981; Fletcher et al., 1996; Max et al., 1998; Max et al., 2004/this issue).

Several additional caveats should be mentioned. First, we had to exclude some children from the analysis of stop-signal task performance because of invalid data. Invalid data indicate that the participant was not fully engaged in the two components of the task, the go and stop tasks. In the presence of invalid data, the assumptions of the race model may not pertain and estimates of SSRT could be inaccurate (Band, 1997; Logan, 1994). A disproportionate number of individuals with invalid performance had severe CHI. Consequently, this method tended to underestimate the extent to which severe CHI was associated with deficient inhibition. Similarly, exclusion of these severe CHI cases may account for the absence of an effect of CHI severity on the speed of response execution. It will be important to develop new methods of assessing response inhibition that will be useful for younger and more impaired children.

Second, we based research diagnoses of SADHD and anxiety on parent and teacher behavior questionnaires. This method does not have the same rigor as a comprehensive clinical diagnostic assessment. Although direct parent and teacher interview would be preferable, we do have confidence in the questionnaire method. For example, we observed that approximately 12% of our control group met criteria for ADHD. This rate is broadly consistent with the general population prevalence of ADHD. Third, we did not sample CHI cases consecutively but enrolled individuals who were willing to participate. This sampling method can introduce a bias in the proportion of cases with preinjury behavior problem, postinjury SADHD, or cognitive difficulties. Prospective samples followed forward are difficult and costly to accrue, but would provide an opportunity to reduce this selection bias and to employ measures of preinjury psychopathology shortly after the injury. A prospective strategy would permit modeling of the interaction over time among the physiological characteristics of head injury, preinjury psychopathology, behavior, and cognitive outcome. Fourth, we had no comparison group of children with injuries other than head injury. This type of control group could help sort out the potential confound of preinjury ADHD in children at risk for injury of any type (Bijur et al., 1988).

CONCLUSION

Bearing these caveats in mind, several conclusions are suggested by these results. This study supports the conclusion that CHI in children can cause SADHD and that severe CHI can cause a syndrome of SADHD and deficient cognitive inhibition. CHI of all degrees of severity predicts development of SADHD symptoms de novo or worsening of preexisting ADHD symptoms. An important finding is that only severe CHI coupled with SADHD was associated with response inhibition deficit. Apparently, less severe CHI does not generate a cognitive phenocopy of ADHD although it can generate a behavioral phenocopy of ADHD. Future research should include a comparison group with primary ADHD unassociated with CHI. The data underscore the importance of cognitive as well as behavioral decomposition of attention disorders from diverse origins.

ACKNOWLEDGMENTS

This research was supported by grants from National Institute for Neurological Disease and Stroke (2R01NS 21889–16) and the Canadian Institutes of Health Research. Jeffrey E. Max was supported by Grant National Institute of Mental Health K–08 MH1800–03.

We acknowledge the assistance of the entire Childhood Head Injury Neurological Outcome team in the collection and coding of data.

REFERENCES

Asarnow, R. F., Satz, P., Light, R., Lewis, R., & Neumann, E. (1991). Behavior problems and adaptive functioning in children with mild and severe closed head injury. *Journal of Pediatric Psychology, 16,* 543–555.

Band, G. P., van der Molen, M. W., & Logan, G. D. (2003). Horse-race model simulations of the stop-signal procedure. *Acta Psychologia, 112,* 105–142.

Barkley, R. A. (1997). Behavioral inhibition, sustained attention, and executive functions: Constructing a unifying theory of ADHD. *Psychological Bulletin, 121,* 65–94.

Barkley, R. A., Guevremont, D. C., Anastopoulos, A. D., DuPaul, G. J., & Shelton, T. L. (1993). Driving-related risks and outcomes of attention deficit hyperactivity disorder in adolescents and young adults: a 3- to 5-year follow-up survey. *Pediatrics, 92,* 212–218.

Barkley, R. A., Murphy, K. R., & Kwasnik, D. (1996). Motor vehicle driving competencies and risks in teens and young adults with attention deficit hyperactivity disorder. *Pediatrics, 98,* 1089–1095.

Bijur, P., Golding, J., Haslum, M., & Kurzon, M. (1988). Behavioral predictors of injury in school-age children. *American Journal of Disease of Child, 142,* 1307–1312.

Bijur, P. E., Stewart-Brown, S., & Butler, N. (1986). Child behavior and accidental injury in 11,966 preschool children. *The American Journal of Disease of Child, 40,* 487–492.

Boyle, M. H., Offord, D. R., Campbell, D., Catlin, G., Goering, P., Lin, E., et al. (1996). Mental health supplement to the Ontario Health Survey: methodology. *The Canadian Journal of Psychiatry, 41,* 549–558.

Boyle, M. H., Offord, D. R., Racine, Y. A., Szatmari, P., Sanford, M., & Fleming, J. E. (1997). Adequacy of interviews vs checklists for classifying childhood psychiatric disorder based on parent reports [see comments]. *Archives of General Psychiatry, 54,* 793–799.

Brown, G., Chadwick, O., Shaffer, D., Rutter, M., & Traub, M. (1981). A prospective study of children with head injuries: III. Psychiatric sequelae. *Psychological Medicine, 11,* 63–78.

Catroppa, C., Anderson, V., & Stargatt, R. (1999). A prospective analysis of the recovery of attention following pediatric head injury. *Journal of International Neuropsychological Society, 5,* 48–57.

Chadwick, O. (1985). Psychological sequelae of head injury in children. *Developmental Medicine and Child Neurology, 27,* 72–75.

Chadwick, O., Rutter, M., Brown, G., Shaffer, D., & Traub, M. U. (1981). A prospective study of children with head injuries: II. Cognitive sequelae. *Psychological Medicine, 11,* 49–61.

Chadwick, O., Rutter, M., Shaffer, D., & Shrout, P. E. (1981). A prospective study of children with head injuries: IV. Specific cognitive deficits. *Journal of Clinical Neuropsychology, 3,* 101–120.

Crosbie, J. M., & Schachar, R. J. (2001). Deficient inhibition as a marker for familial ADHD. *American Journal of Psychiatry, 158* 1884–1890.

Daugherty, T. K., Quay, H. C., & Ramos, L. (1993). Response perseveration, inhibitory control, and central dopaminergic activity in childhood behavior disorders. *Journal of Genetic Psychology, 154,* 177–188.

Dennis, M., Guger, S., Roncadin, C., Barnes, M., & Schachar, R. (2001). Attentional-inhibitory control and social-behavioral regulation after childhood closed head injury: Do biological, developmental, and recovery variables predict outcome? *Journal of International Neuropsychological Society, 7,* 683–692.

Dennis, M., Wilkinson, M., Koski,L., & Humphreys, R. (1995). Attention deficits in the long term after childhood head injury. *Traumatic head injury in children,* 165–187.

Di Stefano, G., Bachevalier, J., Levin, H. S., Song, J. X., Scheibel, R. S., & Fletcher, J. M. (2000). Volume of focal brain lesions and hippocampal formation in relation to memory function after closed head injury in children. *Journal of Neurology, Neurosurgery, Psychiatry, 69,* 210–216.

Eaves, L. J., Silberg, J. L., Meyer, J. M., Maes, H. H., Simonoff, E., Pickles, A., et al. (1997). Genetics and developmental psychopathology: 2. The main effects of genes and environment on behavioral problems in the Virginia Twin Study of Adolescent Behavioral Development. *Journal of Child Psychology & Psychiatry & Allied Disciplines, 38,* 965–980.

Ewing-Cobbs, L., Prasad, M., Fletcher, J. M., Levin, H. S., Miner, M. E., & Eisenberg, H. M. (1998). Attention after pediatric traumatic bran injury: A multidimensional assessment. *Child Neuropsychology, 4,* 35–48.

Filipek, P. A., Semrud-Clikeman, M., Steingard, R. J., Renshaw, P. F., Kennedy, D. N., & Biederman, J. (1997). Volumetric MRI analysis comparing subjects having attention-deficit hyperactivity disorder with normal controls. *Neurology, 48,* 589–601.

Fletcher, J. M., Levin, H. S., Lachar, D., Kusnerik, L., Harward, H., Mendelsohn, D., et al. (1996). Behavioral outcomes after pediatric closed head injury: relationships with age, severity, and lesion size. *Journal of Child Neurology, 11,* 283–290.

Gerring, J. P., Brady, K. D., Chen, A., Vasa, R., Grados, M., Bandeen-Roche, K. J., et al. (1998). Premorbid prevalence of ADHD and development of secondary ADHD after closed head injury. *Journal of the American Academy of Child & Adolescent Psychiatry, 37,* 647–654.

Gordon, M. (1983). *The Gordon Diagnostic System.* DeWitt, NY: Gordon Systems.

Gordon, M. (1988). *The Gordon Diagnostic System: Model III instruction manual.* DeWitt, NY: Gordon Systems.

Herskovits, E. H., Megalooikonomou, V., Davatzikos, C., Chen, A., Bryan, R. N., & Gerring, J. P. (1999). Is the spatial distribution of brain lesions associated with closed-head injury predictive of subsequent development of attention-deficit/hyperactivity disorder? Analysis with brain-image database. *Radiology, 213,* 389–394.

Jennings, J. R., van der Molen, M. W., Brock, K., & Somsen, R. J. (1992). On the synchrony of stopping motor responses and delaying heartbeats. *Journal of Experimental Psychology: Human Perception & Performance, 18,* 422–436.

Jennings, J. R., van der Molen, M. W., Pelham, W., Debski, K. B., & Hoza, B. (1997). Inhibition in boys with attention deficit hyperactivity disorder as indexed by heart rate change. *Developmental Psychology, 33,* 308–318.

Kaufmann, P. M., Fletcher, J. M., Levin, H. S., Miner, M. E., & Ewing-Cobbs, L. (1993). Attentional disturbance after pediatric closed head injury. *Journal of Child Neurology, 8,* 348–353.

Konrad, K., Gauggel, S., Manz, A., & Scholl, M. (2000). Inhibitory control in children with traumatic brain injury (TBI) and children with attention deficit/hyperactivity disorder (ADHD). *Brain Injury, 14,* 859–875.

Kuntsi, J., Oosterlaan, J., & Stevenson, J. (2001). Psychological mechanisms in hyperactivity: I. Response inhibition deficit, working memory impairment, delay aversion, or something else? *Journal of Child Psychology and Psychiatry, 42,* 199–210.

Levin, H. S., Culhane, K. A., Mendelsohn, D., Lilly, M. A., Bruce, D., Fletcher, J. M., et al. (1993). Cognition in relation to magnetic resonance imaging in head-injured children and adolescents. *Archives of Neurology, 50,* 897–905.

Levin, H. S., High, W. M., Jr., Ewing-Cobbs, L., Fletcher, J. M., Eisenberg, H. M., Miner, M. E., et al. (1988). Memory functioning during the first year after closed head injury in children and adolescents. *Neurosurgery, 22,* 1043–1052.

Levin, H., & Kraus, M. F. (1994). The frontal lobes and traumatic brain injury. *Journal of Neuropsychiatry & Clinical Neuroscience, 6,* 443–454.

Levin, H. S., Song, J., Scheibel, R. S., Fletcher, J. M., Harward, H. N., & Chapman, S. B. (2000). Dissociation of frequency and recency processing from list recall after severe closed head injury in children and adolescents. *Journal of Clinical & Experimental Neuropsychology, 22,* 1–15.

Logan, G. D. (1985). On the Ability to Inhibit Simple Thoughts and Actions: II Stop-Signal Studies of Repetition Priming. *Journal of Experimental Psychology, 11,* 675–691.

Logan, G. D. (1994). On the ability to inhibit thought and action: A users' guide to the stop signal paradigm. In D. D. a. T. H. Carr (Ed.), *Inhibitory processes in attention, memory, and language* (pp. 189–239). San Diego, CA: Academic.

Logan, G. D., Cowan, W. B., & Davis, K. A. (1984). On the ability to inhibit simple and choice reaction time responses: A model and a method. *Journal of Experimental Psychology, 10,* 276–291.

Logan, G. D., Schachar, R. J., & Tannock, R. T. (1997). Impulsivity and inhibitory control. *Psychological Science, 8,* 60–64.

Max, J. E., Arndt, S., Castillo, C. S., Bokura, H., Robin, D. A., Lindgren, S. D., et al. (1998). Attention-deficit hyperactivity symptomatology after traumatic brain injury: a prospective study. *Journal of American Academy of Child & Adolescent Psychiatry, 37,* 841–847.

Max, J. E., Lansing, A. E., Koele, S. L. Castillo, C. S., Bokura, H., & Schachar, R. (2004/this issue). Attention deficit hyperactivity disorder in children and adolescents following traumatic brain injury. *Developmental Neuropsychology, 25,* 159–177.

Mendelsohn, D., Levin, H. S., Bruce, D., Lilly, M., Harward, H., Culhane, K. A., et al. (1992). Late MRI after head injury in children: relationship to clinical features and outcome. *Child's Nervous System, 8,* 445–452.

Miller, E. K., & Cohen, J. D. (2001). An integrative theory of prefrontal cortex function. *Annual Review of Neuroscience, 24,* 167–202.

Murray, R., Shum, D., & McFarland, K. (1992). Attentional deficits in head-injured children: An information processing analysis. *Brain & Cognition, 18,* 99–115.

Ollman, R. T. (1973). Simple reactions with random countermanding of the "go" signal. In S. Kornblum (Ed.), *Attention and performance* (Vol. 4, pp. 571–581). New York: Academic.

Oosterlaan, J., Logan, G. D., & Sergeant, J. A. (1998). Response inhibition in AD/HD, CD, comorbid AD/HD + CD, anxious, and control children: A meta-analysis of studies with the stop task. *Journal of Child Psychology & Psychiatry & Allied Disciplines, 39,* 411–425.

Osman, A., Kornblum, S., & Meyer, D. E. (1986). The point of no return in choice reaction time: Controlled and ballistic stages of response preparation. *Journal of Experimental Psychology: Human Perception and performance, 12,* 243–258.

Quay, H. C. (1988). The behavioral reward and inhibition system in childhood behavior disorder. In L. Bloomindale (Ed.), *Attention deficit disorder* (Vol. 3, pp. 176–186). New York: Spectrum.

Quay, H. C. (1997). Inhibition and attention deficit hyperactivity disorder. *Journal of Abnormal Child Psychology, 25,* 7–13.

Robin, D. A., Max, J. E., Steirwalt, J. A. G., Guenzer, L. C., & Lindgren, S. D. (1999). Sustained attention in children and adolescents with traumatic brain injury. *Aphasiology, 13,* 701–708.

Rubia, K., Russell, T., Overmeyer, S., Brammer, M. J., Bullmore, E. T., Sharma, T., et al. (2001). Mapping motor inhibition: Conjunctive brain activations across different versions of go/no-go and stop tasks. *Neuroimage, 13,* 250–261.

Schachar, R., & Logan, G. D. (1990). Impulsivity and inhibitory control in normal development and childhood psychopathology. *Developmental psychology, 26,* 710–720.

Schachar, R., Mota, V. L., Logan, G. D., Tannock, R., & Klim, P. (2000). Confirmation of an inhibitory control deficit in attention-deficit/hyperactivity disorder. *Journal of Abnormal Child Psychology, 28,* 227–235.

Schachar, R., & Tannock, R. (1995). Test of four hypotheses for the comorbidity of attention-deficit hyperactivity disorder and conduct disorder. *Journal of the American Academy of Child & Adolescent Psychiatry, 34,* 639–648.

Schachar, R. J., Tannock, R., & Logan, G. (1993). Inhibitory control, impulsiveness, and attention deficit hyperactivity disorder. *Clinical Psychology Review, 13,* 721–739.

Semrud-Clikeman, M., Filipek, P. A., Biederman, J., Steingard, R., Kennedy, D., Renshaw, P., et al. (1994). Attention-deficit hyperactivity disorder: magnetic resonance imaging morphometric analysis of the corpus callosum. *Journal of the American Academy of Child & Adolescent Psychiatry, 33,* 875–881.

Solanto, M. V. (1990). The effects of reinforcement and response-cost on a delayed response task in children with attention deficit hyperactivity disorder: a research note. *Journal of Child Psychology and Psychiatry, 31,* 803–808.

Solanto, M. V., Abikoff, H., Sonuga-Barke, E., Schachar, R., Logan, G. D., Wigal, T., et al. (2001). The ecological validity of delay aversion and response inhibition as measures of impulsivity in AD/HD: A supplement to the NIMH Multimodal Treatment Study of AD/HD. *Journal of Abnormal Child Psychology, 29,* 215–228.

Teasdale, G., & Jennett, B. (1974). Assessment of coma and impaired consciousness. A practical scale. *Lancet, 2,* 81–84.

Thapar, A., Holmes, J., Poulton, K., & Harrington, R. (1999). Genetic basis of attention deficit and hyperactivity. *British Journal of Psychiatry, 174,* 105–111.

Williams, B., Ponesse, J., Schachar, R., Logan, G. D., & Tannock, R. (1999). Development of inhibitory control across the lifespan. *Developmental Psychology, 35,* 205–213.

DEVELOPMENTAL NEUROPSYCHOLOGY, 25(1&2), 199–225
Copyright © 2004, Lawrence Erlbaum Associates, Inc.

Research on Outcomes of Pediatric Traumatic Brain Injury: Current Advances and Future Directions

H. Gerry Taylor

Department of Pediatrics
Rainbow Babies & Children's Hospital
Case Western Reserve University
Cleveland, Ohio

The articles in this series demonstrate the diversity of research approaches needed to enhance understanding of the sequelae of traumatic brain injury (TBI) in children. Methods ranged from assessment of information processing deficits to evaluation of the construct validity of cognitive tests, tracking of changes in academic achievement after injury, and measurement of behavior and social outcomes. Several articles considered multiple influences on sequelae, including TBI severity, age at injury, time since injury, and preinjury child characteristics. The findings provide new information on injury consequences and the cognitive correlates of postinjury problems in behavior, achievement, and discourse processing. Continued progress requires additional study of relations between specific forms of neuropathology and outcomes, more comprehensive assessments of environmental influences, and greater efforts to monitor postinjury developmental changes. Other needs include more probing assessments of the effects of TBI on daily functioning and social–emotional outcomes, investigation of the specificity of sequelae and of sources of variability in outcome, and application of models that examine mechanisms of effect. This research will benefit clinical practice, clarify processes underlying children's behavior and learning problems, and advance knowledge of normal development.

Children with traumatic brain injury (TBI) have diverse presenting problems (Levin, Benton, & Grossman, 1982). Physical complaints can include headaches, fatigue, dizziness, and disturbances in sensation or sleep. Cognitive symptoms

Requests for reprints should be sent to H. Gerry Taylor, Department of Pediatrics, Rainbow Babies & Children's Hospital, 11100 Euclid Avenue, Cleveland, OH 44106–6038. E-mail: hgt2@po.cwru.edu may involve forgetfulness, slowness and disorganization in completing tasks, word-finding difficulties and other language problems, poor concentration, and inflexible thinking. Problems in behavior and social functioning may be evident in socially inappropriate comments or actions, aggressiveness and temper outbursts, flat affect, apathy, irritability and mood disorders, and lack of insight regarding personal limitations. Symptoms are related in part to TBI severity, age at injury, and time postinjury (Taylor & Alden, 1997). Symptom expression is nevertheless highly variable, even in children and adolescents with serious TBI (Fletcher, Ewing-Cobbs, Francis, & Levin, 1995; Levin, Ewing-Cobbs, & Eisenberg, 1995). Furthermore, some symptoms fail to resolve for years after injury if ever (Klonoff, Clark, & Klonoff, 1993; Thomsen, 1989).

The challenge for the neuropsychologist is to define the presenting problems in behavior, adaptive skills, and learning; explain how these problems come about and why they vary from child to child; and recommend effective interventions (Taylor & Fletcher, 1990). Presenting problems are assessed by obtaining information from children and their parents and teachers. Concerns may include difficulties in getting along with others, following rules and directions, taking tests, and making sound decisions. Behavioral changes observed since the injury are of special interest. The neuropsychologist examines factors that contribute to these problems in several ways: first, by obtaining information about past and current medical status, including the nature of the TBI; second, by reviewing the child's developmental, educational, and family history; and third, by testing cognitive abilities and academic achievement and observing behavior. Test results and observations further define the presenting problems and document cognitive impairments. Other potential influences on presenting problems are assessed by obtaining descriptions of family and school environments and of the child's and family's psychological reactions to the injury. Factors besides TBI that may help account for presenting problems include genetic predispositions to disorders such as learning disabilities or attention deficit hyperactivity disorder (ADHD), behavior or school problems prior to TBI, efforts by the child or others to compensate for weaknesses, symptoms of posttraumatic stress in the child, and injury-related family burden and distress (Asarnow, Satz, Light, Lewis, & Neumann, 1991; Levi, Drotar, Yeates, & Taylor, 1999; Rutter, 1981; Taylor et al., 2001). Although TBI and associated processing deficits may be the major source of presenting problems, all of these factors are considered in establishing etiology. Awareness of problem origins, in turn, guides formulation of treatment plans. Problems that reflect cognitive limitations argue for accommodations or efforts to teach compensatory skills, whereas problems due to behavior mismanagement or motivational issues imply the need for more behaviorally directed treatments. Intervention also entails efforts to avoid or minimize future risks, by suggesting ways to promote educational or social development.

In essence, the neuropsychologist's task is to isolate the "signal" produced by TBI from background "noise," examine reasons for variations in signal characteristics, and integrate this information to formulate probable causes and recommend treatment. Meeting this challenge requires detailed descriptions regarding postinjury deviations in the child's functioning and how problems are manifest at home and school. Because difficulties in behavior or learning are defined relative to age expectations, knowledge of normal development is needed to assess deviancy in outcomes or in developmental trends since the injury. Assessment also entails collection of data on neuropathology, measurement of cognitive deficits that reflect the nature and extent of brain insult, and a theoretical framework for relating these factors to the presenting problems. Recognition of "core deficits" and of how variations in brain pathology map onto these deficits is vital in constructing this framework and in accounting for differences in symptom expression (Dennis, 2000).

Past research on the effects of pediatric TBI has yielded important information on outcomes and risk factors (Yeates, 2000). We have learned that sequelae are variable, but that persisting problems frequently include behavioral disinhibition, memory deficits, slowed response speed, and impairments in perceptual–motor and executive functions. We know that young children are at greater risk for residual impairments and poorer recovery than older children or adolescents (Anderson, Catroppa, Morse, Haritou, & Rosenfeld, 2000; Dennis, Wilkinson, Koski, & Humphreys, 1995; Ewing-Cobbs et al., 1997; Levin et al., 1995). We have also identified injury-related factors that predict outcomes, including the depth and duration of acute postinjury impairments in consciousness and memory (Levin, 1995).

At the same time, past studies have failed to address some of the clinical challenges outlined previously. Little effort has been made to detail presenting problems in children with TBI, or the ways in which these problems vary with contextual demands. Neuropsychological tests have proved poor predictors of key adaptive consequences of injury, such as problems in behavioral self-regulation, school performance, and interpersonal relations (Ewing-Cobbs, Fletcher, Levin, Iovino, & Miner, 1998; Gioia & Isquith, 2004/this issue). Few studies have taken children's preinjury functioning into account, examined changes in sequelae over time postinjury, or evaluated potential moderators of injury effects, such as environmental conditions and the child's age and preinjury characteristics. Although some researchers have examined outcomes in relation to more detailed assessments of brain status (Dennis, Guger, Roncadin, Barnes, & Schachar, 2002; Scheibel & Levin, 1997), many studies continue to rely on a global severity index, such as the Glasgow Coma Scale (GCS) score (Teasdale & Jennett, 1974), as a proxy for degree of neuropathology.

Due in part to the latter limitation and in part to lack of precision in defining neuropsychological sequelae, brain–behavior correlations in children with TBI are not well specified. The central aim of most previous research has been to determine the nature and correlates of sequelae. Few investigations have been designed to test theories of brain–behavior relations, conceptualizations of the origins of postinjury behavior or learning problems, or processes affecting development after TBI. As a result, we are aware of areas of deficits, such as poor school performance and weaknesses in memory and executive function. But we have limited understanding of the neural bases of these impairments, their developmental implications, and how deficits in different domains relate to one another. In addition, there is little consensus regarding how best to conceptualize primary processing deficits or to distinguish these deficits from secondary consequences of injury.

The articles in this issue successfully addressed several of the aforementioned research needs. Many of these articles were the product of interdisciplinary collaborations among researchers from multiple North American sites. As a reflection of this multiplicity, the researchers took a variety of investigational approaches. The methods ranged from factor analysis of neuropsychological measures of executive function (Brookshire, Levin, & Song, 2004/this issue) to assessments of psychosocial disturbances (Gioia & Isquith, 2004/this issue; Max et al., 2004/this issue); tracking of achievement outcomes over time (Ewing-Cobbs et al., 2004/this issue); and experimental manipulations designed to identify specific processing deficiencies in discourse, metacognition, memory, and response inhibition (Chapman et al., 2004/this issue; Hanten et al., 2004/this issue; McCauley & Levin, 2004/this issue; Roncadin, Guger, Archibald, Barnes, & Dennis, 2004/this issue; Schachar, Levin, Max, Chen, & Purvis, 2004/this issue). Despite their differing objectives, each of the articles reflects an interest in broadening the search for determinants of outcome. Examples of this common mind set include investigation of age-related influences on sequelae, preinjury child behavior as a predictor of postinjury attention problems, and the cognitive correlates of problems in behavior, achievement, and discourse macroprocessing. The value of this expanded approach is that it (a) allows for better control of influences on outcomes other than TBI, (b) permits study of moderating effects, and (c) provides clues regarding the nature of the cognitive sequelae of TBI and their implications for children's learning, behavior, and socialization.

The purpose of this commentary is to review the articles in light of current research needs. I first describe the ways in which this series of studies has contributed to measurement of sequelae, appreciation of influences of age-related factors, a broadening of outcome research, and clinical practice. I then consider the methodological strengths and weaknesses of the studies and discuss needs and future directions. Enhanced knowledge of how and why children are adversely affected by TBI, and thus of how to effectively treat them, requires the use of methods that will allow us to better specify and explain injury sequelae.

ADVANCES

Measurement

The most significant contribution of this series of articles is to measurement and conceptualization of deficits in executive function. Deficits in this domain are common among children with TBI, but researchers have only begun to elucidate the dimensions of these problems and their significance in relation to underlying neuropathology and problems in day-to-day functioning (Dennis, Barnes, & Humphreys, 1996; Dennis, Guger, Roncadin, Barnes, & Schachar, 2001; Dennis, Purvis, Barnes, Wilkinson, & Winner, 2001; Scheibel & Levin, 1997). The individual articles focused either on the broader manifestations of executive dysfunction and other cognitive impairments, or on application of newly developed laboratory procedures for fractionating children's executive dysfunctions. Major findings from each of the studies are highlighted below:

1. Factor analyses by Brookshire et al. (2004/this issue) indicated that different tests of executive function placed common processing demands on children with TBI but also confirmed the multidimensional nature of executive functions (Levin, Fletcher, Kufera et al., 1996; Pennington, 1997). Specifically, measures of working memory, set shifting, and allocation of attention loaded separately from response speed and discourse processing.

2. Ewing-Cobbs et al. (2004/this issue) demonstrated that TBI had adverse long-term effects on academic achievement and that these effects were associated with the child's neuropsychological outcomes.

3. Gioia and Isquith (2004/this issue) showed how the recently devised Behavior Rating Inventory of Executive Function (BRIEF) taps variations in behavior that may be inadequately measured by more traditional rating scales. Findings from factor analysis differentiated metacognitive problem solving from behavior regulation, again confirming the multidimensional nature of executive constructs.

4. Max et al. (2004/this issue) documented the utility of formal psychiatric interview schedules in assessing preinjury psychosocial status and detecting novel postinjury behavior disorders.

5. Chapman et al. (2004/this issue) analyzed the manner in which children summarize narratives to determine how TBI affects discourse processing. Their findings suggested that children with TBI had special problems in transforming story content, defined as "the combining of ideas into more concise and generalized statements."

6. McCauley and Levin (2002) found that children with TBI had difficulty relative to controls with orthopedic injuries in "remembering to follow" a previous instruction, confirming weaknesses in prospective memory. Their results also re-

vealed greater effects of prospective memory demands on primary task performance (i.e., slower reaction times) in children with severe TBI than in control children.

7. Roncadin et al. (2004/this issue) examined the nature of working memory deficits in children with TBI. Using a recognition memory task, they separated the ability to store words for later recognition from the ability to maintain performance across trial blocks. Deficiencies were present in both areas in children with severe TBI.

8. Hanten et al. (2004/this issue) found that children with TBI were more prone to overestimate their ability to remember words than were injured controls. However, this difference was observed only for prospective ratings of performance, suggesting impaired metacognitive knowledge. Self-judgments of learning made after the children had engaged in the task failed to discriminate the groups. The children with TBI were also less able than controls to detect anomalies in spoken sentences. The fact that this problem was exacerbated by greater load on working memory provided further evidence for deficits in metacognitive control.

9. Schachar et al. (2004/this issue) also employed an experimental procedure to examine component deficits in children with TBI. Using the stop-signal task paradigm, they measured an inhibitory control process that was distinct from response accuracy or speed. Their findings indicated that children with severe TBI who met criteria for secondary ADHD had a selective impairment in inhibitory control.

Focus on Age Factors and Change

As is fitting given the pediatric focus of this issue, most of the articles considered age-related factors and many assessed skills with protracted periods of development. All of the studies evaluated outcomes several years after injury. Without exception, the findings confirmed chronic sequelae, at least in children with severe TBI. The articles differed widely, however, in their emphasis on age-related differences in outcomes. Hanten et al. (2004/this issue) showed improvements with age in metacognition. Schachar et al. (2004/this issue) considered age at injury, time since injury, and age at assessment on postinjury symptoms of ADHD and performance on the stop-signal task, though they found only age-at-assessment effects. Chapman et al. (2004/this issue) showed that deficits in children with TBI in discourse macroprocessing were greater for children injured prior to 8 years of age than in children injured at later ages. Roncadin et al. (2004/this issue) observed that a younger age at injury and shorter time since injury predicted working memory skills among children with moderate TBI.

Brookshire et al. (2004/this issue) documented relations between an "executive function" factor and adaptive behavior skills 3 years after injury, but not more immediately postinjury. Differences in the sample composition for the earlier versus later assessments, or in reliability of measurement, may have been responsible for this finding. However, these results also raise the possibility of time-lagged sequelae. If present, latent consequences may have reflected either the suppressive influences of executive dysfunction on ongoing development of adaptive behavior or the delayed effects of this dysfunction on later-emerging adaptive skills.

The studies by Schachar et al. (2004/this issue) and Max et al. (2004/this issue) investigated change over time by considering estimates of preinjury behavioral status in analysis of injury effects. They found higher rates of preinjury symptoms of inattention–hyperactivity in children with severe TBI who develop ADHD after injury, suggesting that some children may be more predisposed than others to development of problems in attention and self-control.

Ewing-Cobbs et al. (2004/this issue) examined changes over time more comprehensively than the other studies in this series. In one of the few long-term studies assessing postinjury skill development, these researchers applied growth curve modeling to examine the joint effects of TBI severity and age at injury on changes in academic achievement. They found that younger age at injury predicted slower postinjury progress on tests of arithmetic computations and reading recognition, but that severe TBI was associated with more rapid progress in spelling than was mild-to-moderate TBI. The effects of age at injury are consistent with the less rapid postinjury growth in neuropsychological skills observed in previous studies (Anderson et al., 2000; Ewing-Cobbs et al., 1997; Thompson et al., 1994). The relative increases in spelling among children with severe TBI are also in keeping with research demonstrating greater recovery of function in more severely injured children (Taylor et al., 1999; Taylor et al., 2002; Yeates et al., 1997; Yeates et al., 2002). These results confirm the need to separate recovery of previously developed skills from acquisition of new skills, and they support the hypothesis that early brain insults have time-lagged effects on development (Dennis, 2000; Taylor & Alden, 1997). Study implications would have been clearer if growth differences between the TBI groups (mild–moderate vs. severe) had varied according to age at injury. Inclusion of controls without TBI may have permitted a stronger test of the notion that children injured at young ages show less long-term sparing of function.

Expanded Scope of Inquiry

Fletcher (1988, p. 451) described child neuropsychological approaches as efforts to measure multiple abilities and to relate these abilities to both brain status and child functioning. This series is true to this conceptualization. Relative to the atheoretical approach taken in past research (Brooks, 1984), these studies were more theory driven and broader in scope. Several of the studies explored associations between processing deficits and learning or behavior problems (Brookshire et al., 2004/this issue; Ewing-Cobbs et al., 2004/this issue; Max et al., 2004/this issue; Schachar et al., 2004/this issue). Study findings, together with other recent investigations (Dennis, Guger, et al., 2002), show how knowledge of processing deficits enhances our ability to explain these problems. Other articles examined relations between processing deficits as a means for exploring mechanisms of effect. Chapman et al. (2004/this issue), for example, found that the ability to make narrative transformations was associated with puzzle-solving ability.

Investigation of postinjury deficits in executive function was motivated by hypotheses about the nature of these skills, the neurological systems that subserve them, and their implications for behavioral and social functioning. Research on impairments in discourse processing, prospective memory, working memory, metacognition, and academic achievement was also based on knowledge and theory pertaining to normal and abnormal development of these skills (Chapman et al., 2004/this issue; Ewing-Cobbs et al., 2004/this issue; Hanten et al., 2004/this issue; McCauley & Levin, 2004/this issue; Roncadin et al., 2004/this issue; Schachar et al., 2004/this issue). Max et al. (2004/this issue) widened the search for potential influences on outcomes to include familial dispositions to psychiatric disorders. Although the results failed to confirm these influences on the development of secondary ADHD, this study raises the issue of whether there may be "susceptibility genes" for adverse behavioral outcomes (Plomin & Rutter, 1998).

The "multilevel" approach described by Gioia and Isquith (2004/this issue) further exemplifies this broader explanatory framework. Multilevel methods entail measurements of primary processing deficits, functional outcomes, and environmental systems factors. Study of relations between domains elucidates reasons for the functional impairments, as well as contextual factors that moderate the effects of basic processing deficits on children's functioning. Neuropsychological deficits are appropriately conceptualized both as sequelae of injury and as predictors of other outcomes.

The authors also proposed a useful distinction between the *veridicality* and *verisimilitude* of test constructs. The former term refers to the degree to which a test is capable of predicting problems in behavior and learning, and the latter term to the similarity of test demands to the exigencies of daily life. Greater verisimilitude is likely to enhance the predictive validity of a given measure. Measures that have high verisimilitude may also be useful in pinpointing reasons for failures in functioning in real-life settings, and they permit study of contextual influences in ways not possible with more narrowly defined experimental assessments. In my view, however, tasks with high verisimilitude tap skills contributing to functional impairments rather than child functioning per se. Functional outcomes seem best defined in terms of children's ability to meet societal expectations in key "developmental tasks," including academic achievement, socialization, and rule-governed conduct (Masten & Coatsworth, 1998). Deficiencies in the latter areas are identified by failure to maintain age-expected levels of academic achievement, or by deviancy relative to age standards on assessments of behavior or adaptive skills. If one accepts this conceptual distinction, the BRIEF is best characterized as a measure of functional (i.e., behavior) outcomes.

Relevance for Clinical Practice

The findings from this series have the potential to enhance clinical practice in two ways. First, the assessment procedures are likely to prove useful additions to clinical evaluation of children with TBI. With the exception of the interview techniques employed by Max et al. (2004/this issue) and the published tests and rating scales used in some of the other studies, these procedures are not yet well standardized and require further psychometric study. Nevertheless, the validity of these methods in discriminating children with TBI from uninjured controls, or discriminating mild from severe TBI, suggests that they would have clinical utility in detecting sequelae of TBI and in mapping recovery trends.

Second, by advancing knowledge of the nature of executive dysfunctions and their behavioral manifestations, these studies offer guidance in treating children with TBI. The high incidence of secondary ADHD and the presence of a basic impairment in inhibition underscore the importance of therapies directed at these problems (Gerring et al., 1998). Difficulties in prospective memory, working memory, and maintenance of performance levels over time indicate a need for frequent reminders, efforts to break down task requirements, and pacing (Ylvisaker et al., 2001). Deficiencies in metacognitive knowledge imply that some children with TBI have poor insight about what they know and how quickly they can learn. Children with these sequelae may profit from structured study routines and monitoring to ensure that sufficient time is devoted to new learning. As Chapman et al. (2004/this issue) emphasized, strategy training in text summarization may benefit children with weaknesses in this skill, particulary in light of evidence that these difficulties lead to poor mastery and limited retention of content. The neuropsychologist also needs to be aware of these several deficiencies in administering tests to children with TBI and in interpreting results.

METHODOLOGICAL CRITIQUE

Strengths

In many regards, the articles in this series exemplify sound methodology. Owing to recruitment of participants from multiple sites, the sample sizes for several of the studies were large relative to past standards. In most cases, study designs involved comparison groups of uninjured children or children with orthopedic injuries, and children with TBI were classified according to injury severity. The studies experimentally manipulated task demands and employed factor analytic approaches to clarify deficits and define test constructs (Embretson, 1983). In addition, the researchers used categorical as well as continuous measures of outcome, and both "variable-oriented" and "person-oriented" methods, to study of injury effects

(Masten, 2001). Variable-oriented approaches emphasize relations between variables, such as those between TBI severity and cognitive skills. In contrast, person-oriented methods target individual outcomes of preordained interest (e.g., presence–absence of secondary ADHD), their correlates, and the manner in which they evolve over time. A major virtue of the latter approach is that it allows the researcher to study factors associated with clinically meaningful outcomes.

Limitations

These articles also illustrate three common methodological limitations of research on outcomes of TBI in children. First, assessment of injury characteristics was limited for the most part to the traditional classifications of mild, moderate, and severe TBI as determined by lowest postresuscitation GCS scores, duration of unconsciousness, and presence–absence of neurological abnormalities. Roncadin et al. (2004/this issue) and Max et al. (2004/this issue) localized brain insults. However, the former study defined lesion focus only in terms of the presence versus absence of frontal pathology. Lesion size and location within the frontal lobe were not considered, nor were diffuse injuries taken into account in lesion classification. As the authors pointed out, moreover, neuropathology differed widely for children in the nonfrontal group. The latter study relied on computed tomography (CT) scans to define lesion localization, which are less sensitive in detecting lesions than magnetic resonance imaging (MRI) scans (Scheibel & Levin, 1997). The lack of probing assessments of neuropathology is understandable given that standardized research-grade MRI scans are expensive and not routinely performed. Nevertheless, research employing these methods has identified specific brain–behavior relations in children with TBI (Herskovits et al., 1999; Levin et al., 1997; Scheibel & Levin, 1997). Inclusion of advanced neuroimaging methods would have permitted more fine-grained analysis of relations between injury characteristics and outcomes and may have shed light on the neuropathological correlates of cognitive and behavioral sequelae.

Second, the influences of background child and family factors received insufficient attention. Despite evidence that both preinjury child functioning and the family environment predict outcomes after TBI (Max et al., 1997; Rivara et al., 1994), only three of the studies took one or both of these factors into account in analysis of sequelae (Ewing-Cobbs et al., 2004/this issue; Max et al., 2004/this issue; Schachar et al., 2004/this issue). One reason to consider background factors is to better assess the effects of TBI. Controlling for these influences adjusts for preexisting differences between children with and without TBI or between groups that vary in TBI severity, and it allows for greater precision in measurement of injury effects. Brown, Chadwick, Shaffer, Rutter, and Traub (1981) observed that children with milder forms of TBI have more preinjury behavior problems than do children with severe TBI. Efforts to take preinjury status into account are thus especially important in assessing sequelae of mild TBI. One wonders if the deficits in children with mild TBI demonstrated in three of the studies (Chapman et al., 2004/this issue; Hanten et al., 2004/this issue; McCauley & Levin, 2004/this issue) would have held up had the investigators controlled for background factors, or had they selected comparison groups that were closely matched to the TBI children on these factors. Other reasons for taking background factors into account are to improve accuracy in predicting outcomes and to investigate moderating effects of background factors on injury sequelae (Dennis, 2000; Taylor & Alden, 1997). The presence of problems in learning or behavior before TBI, or a family background characterized by low resources and high stress, increases risks for poor outcomes after TBI. Furthermore, findings by our research group suggest that the negative effects of environmental disadvantage on some outcomes are more pronounced in children with severe TBI than in non–head-injured controls (Taylor et al., 1999; Taylor et al., 2002; Yeates et al., 1997).

Third, with the exception of Ewing-Cobbs et al. (2004/this issue) and Max et al. (2004/this issue), the studies assessed outcomes of TBI at a single point in time several years after injury. Cross-sectional studies advance our understanding of long-term consequences, but are relatively insensitive to the effects of TBI on postinjury development or to changes in sequelae over time (Fletcher et al., 1995; Taylor & Alden, 1997). Because factors related to change may differ from those that predict outcome at any given point in time (Hauser-Cram, Warfield, Shonkoff, & Krauss, 2001), repeated assessments of outcome are needed to understand the developmental implications of TBI. A major disadvantage of cross-sectional designs is that they require the use of between-subjects, rather than within-subjects, comparisons to test for the effects of time since injury. A further disadvantage is that these designs require retrospective sample recruitment. Participants may be more difficult to locate or more reluctant to take part years after injury, introducing possible sampling bias. Assessments of preinjury status may be likewise problematic. Retrospective parent or teacher reports of child status prior to injury are useful if collected soon after injury, but are biased by difficulties in recall if obtained after lengthy postinjury intervals. In addition to avoiding these pitfalls, prospective follow-up designs permit the researcher to preselect specific patterns of change for study, examine the correlates of these patterns, and study relations between changes in the child and changes in the environment (Taylor et al., 2001; Taylor et al., 2002; Yeates et al., 2002).

NEEDS AND FUTURE DIRECTIONS

Advancement of knowledge of pediatric TBI requires that we build on the methodological strengths of these articles and address the aforementioned weaknesses. Progress also demands efforts to overcome measurement limitations, investigate sources of variability in outcomes, examine longitudinal changes in greater depth, and explore the mechanisms that underlie injury consequences. I consider each of these needs in the following.

Measurement Limitations

One critical gap in current knowledge is lack of information as to how children with TBI fall short of expectations placed on them by their parents, teachers, and peers. Research has documented deficiencies in academic achievement and adaptive functioning and higher than normal rates of postinjury grade retention, special education, and behavior and personality changes (Ewing-Cobbs et al., 2004/this issue; Max et al., 2004/this issue). But the "real life" manifestations of these outcomes have not been well characterized. Do problems in classroom learning, for example, reflect difficulty following lectures, organizing or completing schoolwork, understanding concepts, formulating answers, or remembering directions? "Criterion-referenced" methods for evaluating classroom competence, designed to assess the child's ability to participate successfully in the classroom, would reveal demands that are especially problematic for children with TBI and provide new information on injury sequelae. Investigations of reading subprocesses, including speed, phonics skills, and comprehension, have begun to clarify the effects of TBI on academic achievement (Barnes, Dennis, & Wilkinson, 1999). The methods described by Gioia and Isquith (2004/this issue) and Max et al. (2004/this issue) should result in similar refinements in assessment of behavior and social problems. Further efforts at task analysis, direct observation of behaviors and interactions, and assessment of contextual demands are nonetheless needed if we are to appreciate the impact of TBI on daily functioning.

More comprehensive measures of social–emotional outcomes are also needed. Dennis and her colleagues have made strides in defining aspects of social cognition affected by injury, including appreciation of irony and intentionality (Dennis, Purvis, et al., 2001). However, few studies have investigated effects of pediatric TBI on regulation of affect and motivation. Clinical observations of flat affect and the lack of responsiveness to contingent behavior management suggest that these issues are worthy of more in-depth study (Ylvisaker & Feeney, 1995). The effect of frontal lobe insults on social and emotional functioning provides a clear rationale for assessing these outcomes (Eslinger, Biddle, & Grattan, 1997; Rolls, 1999). Other reasons for measuring the effects of TBI on emotions include the positive relation between mastery motivation and rate of cognitive development in children with disabilities (Hauser-Cram et al., 2001), associations between emotional self-regulation and children's cognitive and social competencies (Keating & Miller, 1999; Masten & Coatsworth, 1998), and evidence that emotional processing guides decision making (Bechara, Damasio, & Damasio, 2000). These findings underscore the importance of viewing emotional deficits as primary sequelae of TBI, and of considering the contribution of these deficits to poor judgment, learning problems, and other adverse outcomes of TBI.

A further need is to employ more comprehensive measures of environmental influences. To the extent that environmental factors are considered at all, measurement typically entails only a single index of socioeconomic status. Composites of parent education and occupation, such as the Hollingshead Four Factor Index of Social Status (Hollingshead, 1975), predict child outcomes but provide a limited assessment of the child's environment. Reviews of this topic support use of a wider range of measures (Brooks-Gunn, Duncan, & Britto, 1999; Entwisle & Astone, 1994; Hauser & Warren, 1997). In addition to parent education and occupation, these measures include income, family composition, and neighborhood characteristics. Assessments of the within-family, or "proximal," environment complement measures of "distal" sociodemographic characteristics. Examples of the former measures include assessments of the home environment, social supports and stressors, parent psychological distress, parenting styles, family functioning, and even injury-related family burden (Bendersky & Lewis, 1994; Burgess et al., 1999; Landry, Smith, Swank, & Miller-Loncar, 2000). Evidence that sequelae of TBI are moderated by both proximal and distal family measures also argues for use of multicomponent evaluation of the environment (Taylor et al., 1999; Taylor et al., 2002; Yeates et al., 1997).

A final measurement goal is to place greater emphasis on evaluating the specificity of children's impairments. Distinguishing outcomes that are most affected by injury from those that show relative sparing is essential in defining the boundaries of impairment, searching for causal mechanisms, and designing interventions that capitalize on children's strengths. Several of the articles in this series illustrate the value of this research strategy. Chapman et al. (2004/this issue) found that children with TBI made fewer transformed statements than controls in summarizing a narrative, but that the groups did not differ in terms of untransformed statements. Hanten et al. (2004/this issue) observed that children with TBI had deficits in self-assessments of learning skills prior to task engagement, but not after. Schachar et al. (2004/this issue) reported that children with TBI who had secondary ADHD were impaired in inhibition control, but not in response time. Research to identify and isolate primary cognitive impairments will profit from further efforts to distinguish affected and unaffected outcomes. Based on these findings, candidates for primary deficits include transformational aspects of discourse, use of self-knowledge to inform future actions, and response inhibition.

Analysis of skill discrepancies will be useful in further work to isolate primary deficits. If injury has resulted in a selective impairment, children with TBI should show greater degrees of discrepancy than control children. A related approach is to employ covariance analysis to compare children with and without TBI in an area of deficit, controlling for a skill presumed to be relatively spared by injury. However, the test constructs included in these analyses should be clearly dissociable from one another. Composite measures of ability, like IQ, are less useful than measures of discrete skills. To illustrate, the specificity of a deficit in comprehension of intentionality is more meaningfully defined in relation to another discrete measure of language development, such as vocabulary, than in relation to IQ (e.g., Dennis & Barnes, 2001). The reason for this is that tests of discrete ability will be more likely than an omnibus ability measure to tap separable processing skills. In contrasting deficits with relative strengths, researchers will also need to consider the psychometric properties of their measures (Chapman & Chapman, 1978).

Sources of Variability in Outcome

Much of the heterogeneity of outcomes of TBI is unexplained, even after grouping children into traditional severity classifications. Increased knowledge of the nature and sources of this variability, thus, is another important goal for future research. One strategy for discovering meaningful variations in outcome is to conduct subtype analyses. Subtypes can be identified empirically using cluster analysis (Butler, Rourke, Fuerst, & Fisk, 1997; Donders & Warschausky, 1997) or by a prior subgroupings. Placement of children with TBI into subgroups with and without secondary ADHD illustrates the latter approach (Schachar et al., 2004/this issue; Max et al., 2004/this issue).

A second strategy for identifying sources of heterogeneity is to examine the consequences of specific forms of neuropathology. Studies that have taken this approach show that cognitive and behavioral sequelae of TBI are related to lesion location and depth (Gerring et al., 2000; Herskovits et al., 1999; Levin, 1995; Levin et al., 1993; Levin et al., 1997; Levin, Song, Ewing-Cobbs, & Roberson, 2001). Investigations of the correlates of extent and distribution of diffuse axonal injury, disturbances in cerebral metabolism, and abnormal patterns of cortical activation are promising directions for future research (Bigler, 1999; Scheibel & Levin, 1997). Children's injuries can also be subtyped along multiple dimensions. Roncadin et al. (2004/this issue) took this approach in classifying children according to both TBI severity and frontal pathology. Dennis et al. (1996) employed a similar classification scheme in investigating metacognitive deficits. Subtyping children with mild TBI into subgroups with and without parenchymal insults is another example of this approach (Williams, Levin, & Eisenberg, 1990). To advance knowledge of neuropathological influences on outcomes, researchers can compare groups of children with well-defined differences in neuropathology, examine correspondences between degrees of pathology and outcomes, or conduct single-case studies. Case studies of children with early lesions to discrete regions of the frontal lobe, even if not caused by TBI, have been useful in accounting for variations in behavioral sequelae and in elucidating brain–behavior relations (Anderson, Bechara, Damasio, Tranel, & Damasio, 1999; Eslinger & Biddle, 2000).

A third method for discerning sources of variability in outcome is to sort out primary effects of TBI (i.e., those representing direct effects of brain insult) from indirect consequences. Although we have much to learn about primary deficits, they are exemplified by the core impairments in inhibition, memory processes, and metacognition described in this series. Indirect consequences include secondary effects of these deficits on other mental processes or on behavior, socialization, or academic competence. For example, a core deficiency in working memory may lead to secondary difficulties in other memory processes or in problem solving. Other implications might include poor verbal comprehension of texts or lectures, errors on multistep math problems, or behavioral reactions such as task avoidance or irritability.

These secondary manifestations will depend in part on the severity of the primary deficit, and in part on factors that moderate the expression of that deficit. Assuming that a given core deficit can be reliably detected, its manifestations will vary with the strength of other cognitive skills and coping processes, as well as with levels of environmental supports and demands. Dennis (2000) suggested that some of the variability in impairment after childhood brain insults reflects children's "reserve," a concept referring to the degree to which manifestations of deficits can be buffered or exacerbated by other factors. Dennis further proposed a "threshold theory" that incorporates the concept of reserve and other moderating factors (e.g., age factors, level of challenge involved in the task) to account for variable expression of impairment. The multilevel model described by Gioia and Isquith (2004/this issue) represents a similar approach. To illustrate, a deficit in working memory may have less negative consequences for comprehension of texts in children who have stronger verbal abilities or who have developed compensatory strategies. Similarly, school performance will be more negatively impacted if demands on working memory are high or if teachers fail to accommodate to the deficit.

Explaining the variable manifestations of brain-related deficits, albeit a daunting undertaking, will be facilitated by considering the full range of postinjury changes in the child, and by efforts to identify the sources of variability in different outcomes. The nature of the brain insult may be a major predictor of some outcomes. Other outcomes may be more related to the manner in which the child or family is affected by the traumatic event, the ways in which parents and teachers respond to postinjury difficulties in child functioning, and the child's own capacities for coping with problems or compensating for specific processing deficits (Asarnow et al., 1991).

A general strategy for coming to grips with this complexity is to investigate multiple sources of variance in outcomes, as Ewing-Cobbs et al. (2004/this issue) did in exploring predictors of post-TBI academic achievement. An alternative research strategy is to investigate associations between hypothesized moderator factors and functional disorders in children who share the same primary deficit. An example of this strategy would be to study associations of child and environmental characteristics with symptoms of secondary ADHD in children who have a deficit in inhibition control. Another possibility is to employ path analysis or structural equation modeling to test causal networks that relate primary processing deficits, other child traits, and environmental factors to functional impairments.

Longitudinal Consequences

Existing longitudinal studies provide valuable information on short- and long-term sequelae of TBI (Anderson et al., 2000; Ewing-Cobbs et al., 2004/this issue; Ewing-Cobbs et al., 1997; Ewing-Cobbs et al., 1998; Jaffe, Polissar, Fay, & Liao, 1995; Levin et al., 1995; Levin et al., 1996; Rutter, Chadwick, & Shaffer, 1983; Taylor et al., 1999; Taylor et al., 2002; Yeates et al., 2002). According to these findings, children with moderate and severe TBI make some recovery from initial impairments during the first 1 to 2 years after injury. Recovery is nevertheless incomplete and problems in behavior and school performance are persistent. Recovery gradients and long-term consequences vary across different measures of outcome and are more pronounced in children with severe TBI than in children with mild or moderate injuries. Furthermore, postinjury development is more seriously compromised by injuries during the preschool or early school-age years than by injuries later in childhood.

Despite this knowledge base, we have much to learn about patterns of change after TBI and the processes that underlie that change. Recovery patterns have not been rigorously mapped from initial manifestations of sequelae to their residual forms or resolution. The work of Max and his colleagues in tracking the continuance or resolution of psychiatric sequelae comes closest to this type of investigation (Max et al., 2004/this issue). Notwithstanding the largely descriptive studies of adult outcomes of pediatric TBI (Klonoff et al., 1993; Thomsen, 1989), children have not been followed more than a few years after injury. More rigorous follow-ups into adulthood will clarify long-term rehabilitative needs and improve understanding of how sequelae evolve with age (Dennis, 2000; Eslinger et al., 1997).

Researchers also need to conduct more detailed assessments of the components of change. These components include (a) the degree of initial deficit, (b) the rate of "catch-up" to normative expectations over the first few months or years after TBI, (c) the degree of residual deficit after any short-term gains have leveled off, and (d) longer term changes in the residual deficit (Dennis, 2000; Taylor & Alden, 1997). Study of the nature and correlates of these various components of change is likely to reveal information about distinct developmental processes (Taylor et al., 2002). A pattern of initial impairment followed by resolution or catch-up raises the possibility of neural recovery or reorganization, environmental accommodation, or development of compensatory strategies by the child. A worsening of sequelae with age suggests latent effects of injury, premature arrest of development in the deficit area, or environmental dampening of growth. Even constancy of sequelae over time relative to age appropriate standards has the potential to inform us about growth processes. Stability of deficits with advancing age suggests that TBI can impair a given skill without compromising the process responsible for skill acquisition. An alternative interpretation of cross-age constancy of sequelae is that the abilities of children with TBI fall off over time relative to age expectations, but that the effects of these increasing disparities are offset by growth in compensatory processes.

Other ways to foster progress are to evaluate longitudinal sequelae across a range of outcome measures and consider broader dimensions of change. Relatively steep recovery curves are observed for some outcomes, including sensorimotor status, response speed, perceptual–motor skill, and aspects of expressive language, with lesser gradients of change evident for behavior and school performance (Jaffe et al., 1995; Levin et al., 1982; Levin et al., 1995; Levin et al., 1996; Rutter et al., 1983; Taylor et al., 1999). Dennis, Guger, et al. (2001) reported measure-dependent associations between age-related factors and cognitive outcomes. Ewing-Cobbs et al. (2004/this issue) found differences in patterns and correlates of outcome even within the domain of academic achievement. Study of growth rates for different outcomes will clarify the extent to which effects on development are domain-specific and help distinguish processes underlying short- and long-term changes. Certain changes, for example, may signal resolution of generalized brain dysfunction (e.g., due to edema), whereas other changes may be more reflective of recovery from permanent neural damage or of the impact of environmental factors on development. Some aspects of development may be more negatively affected than others, leading to increasing degrees of discrepancy over time. The implications of differential growth patterns have not been examined in children with TBI, but have been proven useful in accounting for age-related increases in verbal-performance discrepancies in children with Williams syndrome (Jarrold, Baddeley, & Hewes, 1998).

A better understanding of the developmental implications of TBI requires that we assess the impact of a deficit in one area on subsequent changes in other outcomes, explore the effects of TBI on organization of mental abilities, and consider the possibility of different manifestations of the same deficit at different points in development. An example of the first approach would be to determine if early emerging deficits in executive function predict subsequent slowing of social development, or if impairment in preschool language acquisition following TBI in young children predicts academic learning at school age. The need to examine the effects on ability structures is justified by evidence for cortical reorganization following early brain insults and for atypical relations among cognitive skills in children with neurodevelopmental disorders (Fletcher, Brookshire, Landry, & Bohan, 1996; Frith & Happe, 1998; Marin-Padilla, 2000; Oliver, Johnson, Karmiloff-Smith, & Pennington, 2000). To explore these effects, researchers could determine if factor structures of test batteries are similar for children with TBI and uninjured controls, or if factor structures change over time postinjury for children with TBI. Findings by Brookshire et al. (2004/this issue) suggest that skill structures may be less well differentiated immediately after injury than they are after longer follow-up intervals. However, the authors considered only data from children with TBI at the earlier postinjury assessment, whereas they combined data from normal and TBI groups at the later follow-up.

Reasons for examining differential manifestations of deficits across the age range are both substantive and practical. Substantively, it is important to determine if sequelae observed at two disparate ages (e.g., during the first 5 years of life compared to later childhood) reflect the same underlying deficiency—a phenomenon referred to as "heterotypic continuity" (Plomin & Rutter, 1998, p. 1231). The development of tests of specific neuropsychological skills in young children, including measures of preschool executive function, will assist in this effort (Anderson, Catroppa, Morse, & Haritou, 1999; Espy, Kaufmann, Glisky, & McDiarmid, 2001; Korkman, Kirk, & Kemp, 1998). More practically, tests for infants and young children differ markedly in form and content from tests for older children. Following children across age ranges thus involves relating early changes on one test battery to later changes on another set of measures.

As illustrated by Ewing-Cobbs et al. (2004/this issue), growth modeling methods (referred to as multilevel, mixed, or hierarchical linear modeling approaches) offer considerable power and flexibility in analysis of the longitudinal consequences of TBI. These methods have numerous advantages over traditional analysis of variance methods (Burchinal, Bailey, & Snyder, 1994; Francis, Fletcher, Stuebing, Davidson, & Thompson, 1991). They analyze growth as a continuous process over time, rather than in terms of differences, and make use of data from participants with missing observations. They also permit unequal intervals between assessments, model dependencies between repeated assessments, incorporate both continuous and categorical predictors, and allow for inclusion of time-varying covariates. These are major advantages in clinical follow-up studies, in which missing values are difficult to avoid, time between assessments differs across participants or phases of follow-up, and environment influences or other correlates of change vary over time. More recent advances in these techniques make it possible to model changes in latent constructs over time, analyze associations between different types of change, and identify subtypes of change (Collins & Sayer, 2001).

Mechanisms of Effect

A final recommendation is to apply models of cognitive processing, normal and abnormal child development, and brain–behavior relations to guide research efforts and to explore mechanisms of effect. In this issue, Hanten et al. and Roncadin et al. made use of theoretical distinctions between different components of metacognition and working memory to isolate the effects of TBI on this area of competence. Further illustrations of this issue's focus on mechanisms of effect include the following: (a) application of models of normal development and of brain–behavior relations in designing assessment procedures (Chapman et al., 2004/this issue; Gioia & Isquith, 2004/this issue); (b) study of associations among cognitive skills, as Hanten et al. (2004/this issue) did in examining the relation of working memory and metacognition, and as McCauley and Levin (2002) did in exploring the link between prospective memory and response time; and (c) analysis of the cognitive correlates of discourse macroprocessing, academic achievement, and secondary ADHD (Brookshire et al., 2004/this issue; Chapman et al., 2004/this issue; Ewing-Cobbs et al., 2004/this issue; Max et al., 2004/this issue; Schachar et al., 2004/this issue).

Other studies of mechanisms of effect have applied models of frontal lobe function and attention to distinguish different forms of cognitive impairment following pediatric TBI. For example, Levin and his colleagues (Levin et al., 2001; Scheibel & Levin, 1997) found that orbitofrontal lesions predicted errors and rule-breaks on tests of executive functioning, whereas deficits in problem solving ability were more closely associated with dorsolateral frontal lesions or TBI severity. Discovery of differential brain correlates for these contrasting impairments suggest that the impairments are dissociable. Guided by multicomponent models of attention, Anderson, Fenwick, Manly, and Robertson (1998) identified deficits in sustained and divided attention among children with TBI, and Dennis et al. (1995) discovered weaknesses in these children in the ability to inhibit responses to distractors. Correlations between specific types of lesions and attention deficits were not examined in the latter studies, but the findings help to delineate the nature of postinjury attention deficits.

A fuller appreciation of mechanisms of effect will require explanatory frameworks that account for profiles of cognitive ability and disability following TBI in children, associated problems in behavior and learning, and the nature and correlates of postinjury changes in outcome. Models of cognition are exemplified by Pennington's (1994) theory of the separability of frontally mediated working memory and hippocampally mediated long-term memory systems, Dennis's (1991) heuristic for conceptualizing frontal-lobe functions, Roberts and Pennington's (1996) interactive framework for explaining relations between working memory and inhibitory processes, and Barkley's (1997) theory of behavioral inhibition as the basis for deficits in sustained attention and executive function in children with ADHD. Theory-driven structural equation modeling will also be useful in exploring mechanisms of effect on cognition (Taylor, Burant, Holding, Klein, & Hack, 2002).

Disorders in behavior and learning can be investigated by testing models in which specific forms of these disorders are related to distinct types of processing deficits. A primary feature of these models is an attempt to account for heterogeneity in behavior and learning outcomes in terms of the variable effects of TBI on processing skills. Schachar et al. (2004/this issue), for example, found that deficient inhibition control predicts secondary ADHD in children with TBI, but not postinjury anxiety disorders. Analyses by Ewing-Cobbs et al. (2004/this issue) revealed that variations in arithmetic skill in their TBI sample were related to individual differences in spatial memory and perceptual motor ability. Although these studies examine associations within TBI groups, comparisons between children with TBI and children who have other developmental disorders also may be revealing. In a study employing the stop-signal paradigm (Konrad, Gauggel, Manz, & Scholl, 2000), children with TBI exhibited a different pattern of deficits than children with ADHD. Both groups had deficits in inhibition relative to controls, but only the TBI group showed a general slowing of information processing. Future studies comparing children with TBI and children with other conditions may provide additional information on distinct aspects of post-TBI behavior and learning disorders. A further benefit of cross-disorder comparisons is their potential to identify behavior or learning problems that have different origins but share superficial similarities, referred to by Dennis (2000) as "phenocopies."

Models of change after TBI are needed to account for recovery from initial deficits, residual or later-emerging developmental consequences, and effects of age at injury, preinjury child behavior, and environmental factors on outcomes. Recovery can be explained in terms of resolution of secondary brain insults, neural plasticity or reorganization of function, and behavioral compensation (Fletcher, 1988; Nelson & Bloom, 1997; Rutter, 1981). The influences of age at injury and time since injury on outcomes have been attributed to age differences in the effects of TBI on the brain or on neural development, differential effects of brain insult on early versus late-maturing skills, and slowed rates of skill acquisition following TBI (Dennis, 2000; Taylor & Alden, 1997). Unfortunately, these various accounts of postinjury change and age-at-injury effects have not been extensively tested. Even less attention has been paid to mechanisms underlying the influences of preinjury child characteristics and environmental factors on outcomes.

Application of recent advances in neuroimaging and models of developmental processes will help guide future research. Research on recovery, for example, will be facilitated by the use of brain activation methods to investigate reorganization of function following injury (Scheibel & Levin, 1997). Models of development of special relevance in predicting the longitudinal consequences of TBI include Pennington's (1994) integrated theory of cognition and intelligence and Anderson's (1998) theory of minimal cognitive architecture. Pennington's theory hypothesizes that early deficits in a frontally mediated working memory system will limit growth of fluid intelligence more so than growth of crystallized abilities. Anderson's theory proposes two independent mechanisms of knowledge acquisition. The "speed of processing" system underlies individual differences in IQ and is unchanging through development. The "information processing modules" system accounts for changes in cognitive abilities with age and experience and is unconstrained by speed of processing. The latter theory provides a basis for hypothesizing either cross-age constancy of impairment or age-related increases in sequelae, depending on which system has been damaged. Other frameworks for explaining change after TBI are those that consider family influences on development, the role of self-regulatory behaviors in acquisition of social and academic skills, and processes by which children adapt to deficits or environmental risks (Brooks-Gunn et al., 1999; Hauser-Cram et al., 2001; Kay, Newman, Cavallo, Ezrachi, & Resnik, 1992; Keating & Miller, 1999; Landry et al., 2000; Masten, 2001; Masten & Coatsworth, 1998).

CONCLUSION

The neuropsychology practitioner has a substantial fund of knowledge to draw on in assessing children with TBI. Previous research has enlightened us about the types of sequelae to anticipate following injury, the fact that behavior and learning is affected, and predictors of poor outcomes. We know that memory and executive functions are particularly susceptible to injury, that earlier occurring insults and more severe TBI are associated with poorer outcomes, and that preinjury behavior problems and environmental disadvantages pose additional risks for post-injury-onset psychiatric disorders (Fletcher, 1988; Levin et al., 1995; Max et al., 1997; Schwartz et al., 2003). This series of studies adds to this knowledge base by clarifying processing deficits and enhancing understanding of behavioral, achievement, and social outcomes. These studies also provide new information on the cognitive correlates of problems in attention, discourse, and achievement.

Further research is nevertheless needed to advance knowledge of the nature of primary processing deficits and their relations to variations in brain pathology, to better understand factors that influence expressions of these deficits in behavior and learning, and to delineate processes responsible for age-related changes or constancy in sequelae. Progress in this regard will require efforts along several fronts. We must overcome common methodological barriers, including lack of information about brain pathology and failure to follow children prospectively. We must also examine processing deficits and functional disorders in greater detail, while simultaneously broadening the scope of investigation to include studies of multifactorial influences on outcome and of relations between outcome domains. Diverse experimental approaches, information regarding brain–behavior relations, and models of normal and abnormal development will be useful in achieving these aims (Diamond, 1991).

The larger goal of research on pediatric TBI is to elucidate the mechanisms responsible for injury sequelae. Knowledge of the processes most directly affected by brain insult, and of how primary deficits relate to other negative outcomes, will suggest ways to improve assessment techniques and will result in more accurate prediction of injury consequences. A better understanding of how experience affects behavior and influences neural reorganization, and of ways in which children adapt to deficits, will also be useful in designing more effective interventions. In addition to their practical benefits, these research efforts have the potential to shed light on processes underlying behavior and learning disorders associated with conditions besides TBI, and to clarify prerequisites of normal development (Cicchetti & Pogge-Hesse, 1982; Eslinger et al., 1997; Masten, 2001).

ACKNOWLEDGMENTS

The preparation of this article was supported by Grant NS36335 from the National Institute of Neurological Diseases and Stroke.

I thank Maureen Dennis for reviewing the manuscript and making constructive editorial suggestions.

REFERENCES

Anderson, J. M. (1998). Mental retardation, general intelligence and modularity. *Learning and Individual Differences, 10,* 159–178.

Anderson, S. W., Bechara, A., Damasio, H., Tranel, D., & Damasio, A. R. (1999). Impairment of social and moral behavior related to early damage in human prefrontal cortex. *Nature Neuroscience, 2,* 1032–1037.

Anderson, V. A., Catroppa, C., Morse, S. A., & Haritou, F. (1999). Functional memory skills following traumatic brain injury in young children. *Pediatric Rehabilitation, 3,* 159–166.

Anderson, V., Catroppa, C., Morse, S., Haritou, F., & Rosenfeld, J. (2000). Recovery of intellectual ability following traumatic brain injury in childhood: Impact of injury severity and age at injury. *Pediatric Neurosurgery, 32,* 282–290.

Anderson, V., Fenwick, T., Manly, T., & Robertson, I. (1998). Attentional skills following traumatic brain injury in childhood: A componential analysis. *Brain Injury, 12,* 937–949.

Asarnow, R. F., Satz, P., Light, R., Lewis, R., & Neumann, E. (1991). Behavior problems and adaptive functioning in children with mild and severe closed head injury. *Journal of Pediatric Psychology, 16,* 543–555.

Barkley, R. A. (1997). Behavioral inhibition, sustained attention, and executive functions: Constructing a unifying theory of ADHD. *Psychological Bulletin, 121,* 65–94.

Barnes, M. A., Dennis, M., & Wilkinson, M. (1999). Reading after closed head injury in childhood: Effects on accuracy, fluency, and comprehension. *Developmental Neuropsychology, 15,* 1–24.

Bechara, A., Damasio, H., & Damasio, A. R. (2000). Emotion, decision making and the orbitofrontal cortex. *Cerebral Cortex, 10,* 295–307.

Bendersky, M., & Lewis, M. (1994). Environmental risk, biological risk, and developmental outcome. *Developmental Psychology, 30,* 484–494.

Bigler, E. D. (1999). Neuroimaging in pediatric traumatic head injury: Diagnostic considerations and relationships to neurobehavioral outcome. *Journal of Head Trauma Rehabilitation, 14,* 406–423.

Brooks, N. (1984). Cognitive deficits after head injury. In N. Brooks (Ed.), *Closed head injury: Psychological, social, and family consequences* (pp. 44–100). New York: Oxford University Press.

Brooks-Gunn, J., Duncan, G. J., & Britto, P. R. (1999). Are socioeconomic gradients for children similar to those for adults? Achievement and health of children in the United States. In D. P. Keating & C. Hertzman (Eds.), *Developmental health and the wealth of nations: Social, biological, and educational dynamics* (pp. 94–124). New York: Guilford.

Brookshire, B. Levin, H. S., & Song, J. X. (2004/this issue). Components of executive function in typically developing and head-injured children. *Developmental Neuropsychology, 25,* 61–83.

Brown, G., Chadwick, O., Shaffer, P., Rutter, M., & Traub, M. (1981). A prospective study of children with head injuries: III. Psychiatric sequelae. *Psychological Medicine, 11,* 63–78.

Burchinal, M. R., Bailey, D. B., & Snyder, P. (1994). Using growth curve analysis to evaluate child change in longitudinal investigations. *Journal of Early Intervention, 18,* 403–423.

Burgess, E. S., Drotar, D., Taylor, H. G., Wade, S., Stancin, T., & Yeates, K. O. (1999). The Family Burden of Injury Interview: Reliability and validity studies. *Journal of Head Trauma Rehabilitation, 14,* 394–405.

Butler, K., Rourke, B. P., Fuerst, D. R., & Fisk, J. L. (1997). A typology of psychosocial functioning in pediatric closed head injury. *Child Neuropsychology, 3,* 98–133.

Chapman, L. J., & Chapman, J. P. (1978). The measurement of differential deficit. *Journal of Psychiatry Research, 14,* 303–311.

Chapman, S. B., Sparks, G., Levin, H. S., Dennis, M., Roncadin, C., Zhang, L., et al. (2004/this issue). Discourse macrolevel processing after severe pediatric traumatic brain injury. *Developmental Neuropsychology, 25,* 37–60.

Cicchetti, D., & Pogge-Hess, P. (1982). Possible contributions of the study of organically retarded persons to developmental theory. In E. Zigler & D. Balla (Eds.), *Mental retardation: The developmental-difference controversy* (pp. 277–318). Hillsdale, NJ: Lawrence Erlbaum Associates, Inc.

Collins, L. M., & Sayer, A. G. (2001). *New methods for the analysis of change.* Washington, DC: American Psychological Association.

Dennis, M. (1991). Frontal lobe function in childhood and adolescence: A heuristic for assessing attention regulation, executive control, and the intentional states important for social discourse. *Developmental Neuropsychology, 7,* 327–358.

Dennis, M. (2000). Childhood medical disorders and cognitive impairment: Biological risk, time, development, and reserve. In K. O. Yeates, M. D. Ris, & H. G. Taylor (Eds.), *Pediatric neuropsychology: Research, theory, and practice* (pp. 3–22). New York: Guilford.

Dennis, M., & Barnes, M. A. (2001). Comparison of literal, inferential, and intentional text comprehension in children with mild or severe closed head injury. *Journal of Head Trauma Rehabilitation, 16,* 456–468.

Dennis, M., Barnes, M. A., & Humphreys, R. P. (1996). Appraising and managing knowledge: Metacognitive skills after childhood head injury. *Developmental Neuropsychology, 12,* 77–103.

Dennis, M., Guger, S., Roncadin, C., Barnes, M., & Schachar, R. (2001). Attentional-inhibitory control and social-behavioral regulation after childhood closed head injury: Do biological, developmental, and recovery variables predict outcome? *Journal of the International Neuropsychological Society, 7,* 683–692.

Dennis, M., Purvis, K., Barnes, M. A., Wilkinson, M., & Winner, E. (2001). Understanding literal truth, ironic criticism, and deceptive praise following childhood head injury. *Brain and Language, 76.*

Dennis, M., Wilkinson, M., Koski, L., & Humphreys, R. P. (1995). Attention deficits in the long term after childhood head injury. In S. H. Broman & M. E. Michel (Eds.), *Traumatic head injury in children* (pp. 165–187). New York: Oxford University Press.

Diamond, A. (1991). Guidelines for the study of brain-behavior relationships during development. In H. S. Levin, H. M. Eisenberg, & A. L. Benton (Eds.), *Frontal lobe function and dysfunction* (pp. 339–378). New York: Oxford University Press.

Donders, J., & Warschausky, S. (1997). WISC-III factor patterns after traumatic head injury in children. *Child Neuropsychology, 3,* 71–78.

Embretson, S. (1983). Construct validity: Construct representation versus nomothetic span. *Psychological Bulletin, 93,* 179–197.

Entwisle, D. R., & Astone, N. M. (1994). Some practical guidelines for measuring youth's race/ethnicity and socioeconomic status. *Child Development, 65,* 1521–1540.

Eslinger, P. J., & Biddle, K. R. (2000). Adolescent neuropsychological development after early right prefrontal cortex damage. *Developmental Neuropsychology, 18,* 297–329.

Eslinger, P. J., Biddle, K. R., & Grattan, L. M. (1997). Cognitive and social development in children with prefrontal cortex lesions. *Development of the prefrontal cortex: Evolution, neurobiology, and behavior* (pp. 295–335). Baltimore: Brookes.

Espy, K. A., Kaufmann, P. M., Glisky, M. L., & McDiarmid, M. D. (2001). New procedures to assess executive functions in preschool children. *The Clinical Neuropsychologist, 15,* 46–58.

Ewing-Cobbs, L., Barnes, M., Fletcher, J. M., Levin, H. S., Swank, P. R., & Song, J. (2004/this issue). Modeling of longitudinal academic achievement scores after pediatric traumatic brain injury. *Developmental Neuropsychology, 25,* 107–133.

Ewing-Cobbs, L., Fletcher, J. M., Levin, H. S., Francis, D. J., Davidson, K., & Miner, M. E. (1997). Longitudinal neuropsychological outcome in infants and preschoolers with traumatic brain injury. *Journal of the International Neuropsychological Society, 3,* 581–591.

Ewing-Cobbs, L., Fletcher, J. M., Levin, H. S., Iovino, I., & Miner, M. E. (1998). Academic achievement and academic placement following traumatic brain injury in children and adolescents: A two-year longitudinal study. *Journal of Clinical and Experimental Neuropsychology, 20,* 769–781.

Fletcher, J. M. (1988). Brain-injured children. In E. J. Mash & L. G. Terdal (Eds.), *Behavioral assessment of childhood disorders* (pp. 451–488). New York: Guilford.

Fletcher, J. M., Brookshire, B., Landry, S. H., & Bohan, T. P. (1996). Attentional skills and executive functions in children with early hydrocephalus. *Developmental Neuropsychology, 12,* 53–76.

Fletcher, J. M., Ewing-Cobbs, L., Francis, D. J., & Levin, H. S. (1995). Variability in outcomes after traumatic brain injury in children: A developmental perspective. In S. H. Broman & M. E. Michel (Eds.), *Traumatic head injury in children* (pp. 3–21). New York: Oxford University Press.

Francis, D. J., Fletcher, J. M., Stuebing, K. K., Davidson, K. C., & Thompson, N. M. (1991). Analysis of change: Modeling individual growth. *Journal of Consulting and Clinical Psychology, 59,* 27–37.

Frith, U., & Happe, F. (1998). Why specific developmental disorders are not specific: On-line and developmental effects in autism and dyslexia. *Developmental Science, 1,* 267–272.

Gerring, J. P., Brady, K., Chen, A., Quinn, C., Herskovitz, E., Bandeen-Roche, K., et al. (2000). Neuroimaging variables related to development of secondary attention deficit hyperactivity disorder after closed head injury in children and adolescents. *Brain Injury, 14,* 205–218.

Gerring, J. P., Brady, K. D., Chen, A., Vasa, R., Grados, M., Bandeen-Roche, K., et al. (1998). Premorbid prevalence of ADHD and development of secondary ADHD after closed head injury. *Journal of the American Academy of Child and Adolescent Psychiatry, 37,* 647–654.

Gioia, G. A., & Isquith, P. K. (2004/this issue). Ecological assessment of executive function in traumatic brain injury. *Developmental Neuropsychology, 25,* 135–158.

Hanten, G., Dennis, M., Zhang, L., Barnes, M., Roberson, G., Archibald, J., et al. (2004/this issue). Childhood head injury and metacognitive processes in language and memory. *Developmental Neuropsychology.*

Hauser, R. M., & Warren, J. R. (1997). Socioeconomic indexes for occupations: A review, update, and critique. In A. E. Raftery (Ed.), *Sociological methodology* (pp. 177–298). Cambridge, MA: Basil Blackwell.

Hauser-Cram, P., Warfield, M. E., Shonkoff, J. P., & Krauss, M. W. (2001). Children with disabilities: A longitudinal study of child development and parent well-being. *Monographs of the Society for Research in Child Development, 66,* Serial No. 266.

Herskovits, E. H., Megalooikonomou, C. D., Davatzikos, C., Chen, A., Bryan, R. N., & Gerring, J. P. (1999). Is the spatial distribution of brain lesions associated with closed-head injury predictive of

subsequent development of attention-deficit/hyperactivity disorder? Analysis with brain-image database. *Radiology, 213,* 389–394.

Hollingshead, A. (1975). *Four Factor Index of Social Status.* New Haven, CT: Yale University.

Jaffe, K. M., Polissar, N. L., Fay, G. C., & Liao, S. (1995). Recovery trends over three years following
pediatric traumatic brain injury. *Archives of Physical Medicine and Rehabilitation, 76,* 17–26.

Jarrold, C., Baddeley, A. D., & Hewes, A. K. (1998). Verbal and nonverbal abilities in the Williams
Syndrome phenotype: Evidence for diverging developmental trajectories. *Journal of Child Psychology and Psychiatry, 39,* 511–523.

Kay, T., Newman, B., Cavallo, M., Ezrachi, O., & Resnik, M. (1992). Toward a
neuropsychological model of functional disability after mild traumatic brain injury.
Neuropsychology, 6, 371–384.

Keating, D. P., & Miller, F. K. (1999). Individual pathways in competence and coping: From regulatory
systems to habits of mind. In D. P. Keating & C. Hertzman (Eds.), *Developmental health and the
wealth of nations: Social, biological, and educational dynamics* (pp. 220–233). New York: Guilford.

Klonoff, H., Clark, C., & Klonoff, P. S. (1993). Long-term outcome of head injuries: A 23 year follow-up study of children with head injuries. *Journal of Neurology, Neurosurgery, and Psychiatry, 56,*
410–415.

Konrad, K., Gauggel, S., Manz, A., & Scholl, M. (2000). Inhibitory control in children with traumatic
brain injury (TBI) and children with attention deficit/hyperactivity disorder (ADHD). *Brain Injury,
14,* 859–875.

Korkman, M., Kirk, U., & Kemp, S. (1998). *NEPSY: A Developmental Neuropsychological Assessment, manual.* San Antonio, TX: Psychological Corporation.

Landry, S. H., Smith, K. E., Swank, P. R., & Miller-Loncar, C. L. (2000). Early maternal and child influences on children's later independent cognitive and social functioning. *Child Development, 71,*
358–375.

Levi, R. B., Drotar, D., Yeates, K. O., & Taylor, H. G. (1999). Posttraumatic stress symptoms in children following orthopedic or traumatic brain injury. *Journal of Clinical Child Psychology, 28,*
232–243.

Levin, H. S. (1995). Prediction of recovery from traumatic brain injury. *Journal of Neurotrauma, 12,*
913–922.

Levin, H. S., Benton, A. L., & Grossman, R. G. (1982). *Neurobehavioral consequences of closed head
injury.* New York: Oxford University Press.

Levin, H. S., Culhane, K. A., Mendelsohn, D., Lilly, M. A., Bruce, D., Fletcher, J. M., et al. (1993).
Cognition in relation to magnetic resonance imaging in head-injured children and adolescents. *Archives of Neurology, 50,* 897–905.

Levin, H. S., Ewing-Cobbs, L., & Eisenberg, H. M. (1995). Neurobehavioral outcome of pediatric
closed head injury. In S. H. Broman & M. E. Michel (Eds.), *Traumatic head injury in children* (pp.
70–94). New York: Oxford University Press.

Levin, H. S., Fletcher, J. M., Kusnerik, L., Kufera, J. A., Lilly, M. A., Duffy, F. F., et al. (1996). Semantic memory following pediatric head injury: Relationship to age, severity of injury, and MRI. *Cortex,
32,* 461–478.

Levin, H. S., Mendelsohn, D., Lilly, M. A., Yeakley, J., Song, J., Scheibel, R. S., et al. (1997). Magnetic
resonance imaging in relation to functional outcome of pediatric closed head injury: A test of the
Ommaya-Gennarelli Model. *Neurosurgery, 40,* 432–441.

Levin, H. S., Song, J., Ewing-Cobb, L., & Roberson, G. (2001). Porteus maze performance following
traumatic brain injury in children. *Neuropsychology, 15,* 557–567.

Marin-Padilla, M. (2000). Perinatal brain damage, cortical reorganization (acquired cortical
dysplasias), and epilepsy. In P. D. Williamson, A. M. Siegel, D. W. Roberts, M. V. Thadani, & M. S.
Gazzaniga, M. S. (Eds.), *Neocortical epilepsies: Advances in neurology* (Vol. 84, pp. 153–172). Philadelphia: Lippincott.

Masten, A. S. (2001). Ordinary magic: Resilience processes in development. *American Psychologist, 56,* 227–238.

Masten, A. S., & Coatsworth, J. D. (1998). The development of competence in favorable and unfavorable environments: Lessons from research on successful children. *American Psychologist, 53,* 204–220.

Max, J. E., Lansing, A. E., Koele, S. L., Castillo, C. C., Bokura, H., Collings, N., et al. (2004/this issue). Attention deficit hyperactivity disorder in children and adolescents following traumatic brain injury. *Developmental Neuropsychology, 25,* 159–177.

Max, J. E., Robin, D. A., Lindgren, S. D., Smith, W. L., Jr., Sato, Y., Mattheis, P. J., et al. (1997). Traumatic brain injury in children and adolescents: Psychiatric disorders at two years. *Journal of the American Academy of Child and Adolescent Psychiatry, 36,* 1278–1285.

McCauley, S. R., & Levin, H. S. (2004/this issue). Prospective memory in pediatric traumatic brain injury: A preliminary study. *Developmental Neuropsychology, 25,* 5–20.

Nelson, C. A., & Bloom, F. E. (1997). Child development and neuroscience. *Child Development, 68,* 970–987.

Oliver, A., Johnson, M. H., Karmiloff-Smith, A., & Pennington, B. (2000). Deviations in the emergence of representations: A neuroconstructivist framework for analysing developmental disorders. *Developmental Science, 3,* 1–40.

Pennington, B. F. (1994). The working memory function of the prefrontal cortices: Implications for developmental and individual differences in cognition. In M. M. Haith, J. Benson, R. Roberts, & B. F. Pennington (Eds.), *The development of future oriented processes* (pp. 243–289). Chicago: University of Chicago Press.

Pennington, B. F. (1997). Dimensions of executive functions in normal and abnormal development. In N. A. Krasnegor, G. R. Lyon, & P. S. Goldman-Rakic, P. S. (Eds.), *Development of the prefrontal cortex: Evolution, neurobiology, and behavior* (pp. 265–281). Baltimore: Brookes.

Plomin, R., & Rutter, M. (1998). Child development, molecular genetics, and what to do with genes once they are found. *Child Development, 69,* 1223–1242.

Rivara, J. B., Jaffe, K. M., Polissar, N. L., Fay, G. C., Martin, K. M., Shurtleff, H. A., et al. (1994). Family functioning and children's academic performance and behavior problems in the year following traumatic brain injury. *Archives of Physical Medicine and Rehabilitation, 75,* 369–379.

Roberts, R. J., Jr., & Pennington, B. F. (1996). An interactive framework for examining prefrontal cognitive processes. *Developmental Neuropsychology, 12,* 105–126.

Rolls, E. T. (1999). *The brain and emotion.* Oxford, England: Oxford University Press.

Roncadin, C., Guger, S., Archibald, J., Barnes, M., & Dennis, M. (2004/this issue). Working memory after childhood closed head injury. *Developmental Neuropsychology, 25,* 21–36.

Rutter, M. (1981). Psychological sequelae of brain damage in children. *American Journal of Psychiatry, 138,* 1533–1544.

Rutter, M., Chadwick, O., & Shaffer, D. (1983). Head injury. In M. Rutter (Ed.), *Developmental psychiatry* (pp. 83–111). New York: Guilford.

Schachar, R., Levin, H. S., Max, J., Chen, S., & Purvis, K. (2004/this issue). Attention deficit hyperactivity disorder and inhibition deficit after closed head injury in children: Do preinjury behavior, injury severity, and recovery variables predict outcome? *Developmental Neuropsychology, 25,* 179–198.

Scheibel, R. S., & Levin, H. S. (1997). Frontal lobe dysfunction following closed head injury in children: Findings from neuropsychology and brain imaging (pp. 241–263). In N. A. Krasnegor, G. R. Lyon, & P. S. Goldman-Rakic (Eds.), *Development of the prefrontal cortex: Evolution, neurobiology, and behavior* (pp. 265–281). Baltimore: Brookes.

Schwartz, L., Taylor, H. G., Drotar, D., Yeates, K. O., Wade, S. L., & Stancin, T. (2003). Long-term behavior problems after pediatric traumatic brain injury: Prevalence, predictors, and correlates. *Journal of Pediatric Psychology, 28,* 251–264.

Taylor, H. G., & Alden, J. (1997). Age-related differences in outcomes following childhood brain insults: An introduction and overview. *Journal of the International Neuropsychological Society, 3,* 555–567.

Taylor, H. G., Burant, C., Holding, P. A., Klein, N., & Hack, M. (2002). Sources of variability in sequelae of very low birth weight. *Child Neuropsychology, 8,* 163–178.

Taylor, H. G. & Fletcher J. M. (1990). Neuropsychological assessment of children. In M. Hersen & G. Goldstein (Eds.), *Handbook of psychological assessment* (2nd ed., pp. 228–255). New York: Plenum.

Taylor, H. G., Yeates, K. O., Wade, S. L., Drotar, D., Stancin, T., & Burant, C. (2001). Bidirectional child-family influences on outcomes of traumatic brain injury in children. *Journal of the International Neuropsychological Society, 7,* 755–767.

Taylor, H. G., Yeates, K. O., Wade, S. L., Drotar, D., Stancin, T., & Klein, S. (1999). Influences on first-year recovery from traumatic brain injury in children. *Neuropsychology, 13,* 76–89.

Taylor, H. G., Yeates, K. O., Wade, S. L., Drotar, D., Stancin, T., & Minich, N. (2002). A prospective study of long- and short-term outcomes after traumatic brain injury in children: Behavior and achievement. *Neuropsychology, 16,* 15–27.

Teasdale, G., & Jennett, B. (1974). Assessment of coma and impaired consciousness: A practical scale. *Lancet, 2,* 81–84.

Thompson, N. M., Francis, D. J., Stuebing, K. K., Fletcher, J. M., Ewing-Cobbs, L., Miner, M. E., et al. (1994). Motor, visual-spatial, and somatosensory skills after closed head injury in children and adolescents: A study of change. *Neuropsychology, 8,* 333, 342.

Thomsen, I. V. (1989). Do young patients have worse outcomes after severe blunt head trauma? *Brain Injury, 3,* 157–162.

Williams, D. H., Levin, H. S., & Eisenberg, H. M. (1990). Mild head injury classification. *Neurosurgery, 27,* 422–428.

Yeates, K. O. (2000). Closed-head injury. In K. O. Yeates, M. D. Ris, & H. G. Taylor (Eds.), *Pediatric neuropsychology: Research, theory, and practice* (pp. 922–116). New York: Guilford.

Yeates, K. O., Taylor, H. G., Drotar, D., Wade, S. L., Stancin, T., & Klein, S. (1997). Preinjury family environment as a determinant of recovery from traumatic brain injury in school-age children. *Journal of the International Neuropsychological Society, 3,* 617–630.

Yeates, K. O., Taylor, H. G., Wade, S. L., Drotar, D., Stancin, T., & Minich, N. (2002). A prospective study of short- and long-term neuropsychological outcomes after traumatic brain injury in children. *Neuropsychology, 16,* 514–523.

Ylvisaker, M., & Feeney, T. J. (1995). Traumatic brain injury in adolescence: Assessment and reintegration. *Seminars in Speech and Language, 16,* 32–44.

Ylvisaker, M., Todis, B., Glang, A., Urbanczyk, B., Franklin, C., DePompei, R., et al. (2001). Educating students with TBI: Themes and recommendations. *Journal of Head Trauma Rehabilitation, 16,* 76–93.

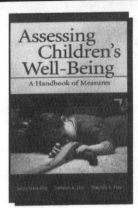

2004 SUBSCRIPTION ORDER FORM

Please ❑ enter ❑ renew my subscription to:

DEVELOPMENTAL NEUROPSYCHOLOGY

AN INTERNATIONAL JOURNAL OF LIFE-SPAN ISSUES IN NEUROPSYCHOLOGY

Volume 25 & 26, 2004, 6 Issues — ISSN 8756–5641/Online ISSN 1532–6942

SUBSCRIPTION PRICES PER VOLUME:

Category:	Access Type:	Price: US-Canada/All Other Countries
❑ Individual	Online & Print	$100.00/$145.00

Subscriptions are entered on a calendar-year basis only and must be paid in advance in U.S. currency—check, credit card, or money order. Prices for subscriptions include postage and handling. **Journal prices expire 12/31/04.** NOTE: Institutions must pay institutional rates. Individual subscription orders are welcome if prepaid by credit card or personal check. **Please note:** A $20.00 penalty will be charged against customers providing checks that must be returned for payment. This assessment will be made only in instances when problems in collecting funds are directly attributable to customer error.

❑ **Check Enclosed** (U.S. Currency Only)   **Total Amount Enclosed $**_____

❑ **Charge My:** ❑ VISA   ❑ MasterCard   ❑ AMEX   ❑ Discover

Card Number _____   Exp. Date_____/_____

Signature_____
(Credit card orders cannot be processed without your signature.)
PRINT CLEARLY for proper delivery. STREET ADDRESS/SUITE/ROOM # REQUIRED FOR DELIVERY.

Name_____

Address_____

City/State/ Zip+4_____

Daytime Phone #_____E-mail address_____
Prices are subject to change without notice.

For information about online subscriptions, visit our website at *www.erlbaum.com*

Mail orders to: **Lawrence Erlbaum Associates, Inc.,** Journal Subscription Department
10 Industrial Avenue, Mahwah, NJ 07430; **(201) 258–2200;** FAX **(201) 760–3735; journals@erlbaum.com**

LIBRARY RECOMMENDATION FORM

Detach and forward to your librarian.

❑ I have reviewed the description of *Developmental Neuropsychology* and would like to recommend it for acquisition.

DEVELOPMENTAL NEUROPSYCHOLOGY

AN INTERNATIONAL JOURNAL OF LIFE-SPAN ISSUES IN NEUROPSYCHOLOGY

Volume 25 & 26, 2004, 6 Issues — ISSN 8756–5641/Online ISSN 1532–6942

Category:	Access Type:	Price: US-Canada/All Other Countries
❑ Institutional	Online & Print	$825.00/$870.00
❑ Institutional	Online Only	$700.00/$700.00
❑ Institutional	Print Only	$745.00/$790.00

Name_____Title_____

Institution/Department_____

Address_____

E-mail Address_____
Librarians, please send your orders directly to LEA or contact from your subscription agent.

Lawrence Erlbaum Associates, Inc., Journal Subscription Department
10 Industrial Avenue, Mahwah, NJ 07430; **(201) 258–2200;** FAX **(201) 760–3735; journals@erlbaum.com**

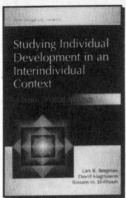

STUDYING INDIVIDUAL DEVELOPMENT IN AN INTERINDIVIDUAL CONTEXT

A Person-Oriented Approach

Lars R. Bergman
David Magnusson
Bassam M. El Khouri

Stockholm University

During the last decade there has been increased awareness of the limitations of standard approaches to the study of development. When the focus is on variables and relationships, the individual is easily lost.

This book describes an alternative, person-oriented approach in which the focus is on the individual as a functioning whole. The authors take as their theoretical starting points the holistic-interactionistic research paradigm expounded by David Magnusson and others, and the new developmental science in which connections and interactions between different systems (biological, psychological, social, etc.) are stressed. They present a quantitative methodology for preserving—to the maximum extent possible—the individual as a functioning whole that is largely based on work carried out in the Stockholm Laboratory for Developmental Science over the past 20 years.

The book constitutes a complete introductory guide to the person-oriented approach. The authors lay out the underlying theory, a number of basic methods, the necessary computer programs, and an extensive empirical example. (The computer programs have been collected into a statistical package, SLEIPNER, that is freely accessible on the Internet. The empirical example deals with boys' school adjustment from a pattern perspective and covers both positive and negative adaptation.)

Studying Individual Development in an Interindividual Context: A Person-Oriented Approach will be crucial reading for all researchers who seek to understand the complexities of human development and for their advanced students.

Contents: Preface. Introduction. Theoretical Framework. General Methodological Considerations. Classification in a Person-Oriented Context. Analyzing All Possible Patterns. Some Methods for Studying Pattern Development. Examining the Generalizability of Results. SLEIPNER, A Statistical Package for Person-Oriented Analysis. Stability and Change in Patterns of School Adjustment: An Empirical Study. Discussion and Directions.
0-8058-3129-0 [cloth] / 2003 / 232pp. / $49.95
0-8058-3130-4 [paper] / 2003 / 232pp. / $27.50
Prices are subject to change without notice.

Lawrence Erlbaum Associates, Inc.

10 Industrial Ave., Mahwah, NJ 07430–2262
201–258–2200; 1–800–926–6579; fax 201–760–3735
orders@erlbaum.com; www.erlbaum.com

PSYCHOPHYSICS BEYOND SENSATION

Laws and Invariants of Human Cognition

Edited by

Christian Kaernbach
Erich Schröger
University of Leipzig, Germany
Hermann Müller
Ludwig-Maximilians-Universität, München Germany
and *University of London, UK*
A Volume in the Scientific Psychology Series

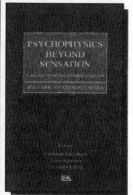

This volume presents a series of studies that expand laws, invariants, and principles of psychophysics beyond its classical domain of sensation. In spite of the equivalence of methods, such contributions are often not regarded as "psychophysics." This book's goal is to demonstrate the extent of the domain of psychophysics, ranging from sensory processes, through sensory memory and short-term memory issues, to the interaction between sensation and action. The dynamics and timing of human performance are a further important issue within this extended framework of psychophysics: Given the similarity of the various cortical areas in terms of their neuroanatomical structure, it is an important question whether this similarity is paralleled by a similarity of processes. These issues are addressed by the contributions in the present volume using state-of-the-art research methods in behavioral research, psychophysiology, and mathematical modeling.

The book is divided into four sections. Part I presents contributions concerning the classical domain of psychophysical judgment. The next two parts are concerned with elementary and higher-order processes and the concluding section deals with psychophysical models. The sections are introduced by guest editorials contributed by independent authors. These editorials present the authors' personals view on the respective section, providing an integrated account of the various contributions or highlighting their focus of interest among them. While also voicing their own and sometimes different point of view, they contribute to the process of discussion that makes science so exciting.

This volume should be of great interest to advanced students in neuroscience, cognitive science, psychology, neuropsychology, and related areas who seek to evaluate the range and power of psychological work today. Established scientists in those fields will also appreciate the variety of issues addressed within the same methodological framework and their multiple interconnections and stimulating "cross-talk."

0-8058-4250-0 [cloth] / 2004 / 544pp. / $135.00

Special Discount Price! $60.00

Applies if payment accompanies order or for course adoption orders of 5 or more copies. **No further discounts apply.**
Prices are subject to change without notice.

Lawrence Erlbaum Associates, Inc.

10 Industrial Ave., Mahwah, NJ 07430–2262
201–258–2200; 1–800–926–6579; fax 201–760–3735
orders@erlbaum.com; www.erlbaum.com

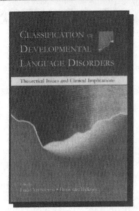

CLASSIFICATION OF DEVELOPMENTAL LANGUAGE DISORDERS

Theoretical Issues and Clinical Implications

Edited by

Ludo Verhoeven
Hans van Balkom
University of Nijmegen

Chapters written by leading authorities offer current perspectives on the origins and development of language disorders. They address the question: How can the child's linguistic environment be restructured so that children at risk can develop important adaptive skills in the domains of self-care, social interaction, and problem solving? This theory-based, but practical book emphasizes the importance of accurate definitions of subtypes for assessment and intervention. It will be of interest to students, researchers, and practitioners in the field of developmental language disorders.

0-8058-4122-9 [cloth] / 2004 / 464pp. / $99.95
0-8058-4123-7 [paper] / 2004 / 464pp. / $49.95
Prices are subject to change without notice.

Lawrence Erlbaum Associates, Inc.
10 Industrial Ave., Mahwah, NJ 07430–2262
201–258–2200; 1–800–926–6579; fax 201–760–3735
orders@erlbaum.com; www.erlbaum.com

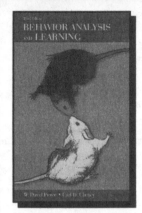

BEHAVIOR ANALYSIS AND LEARNING

Third Edition
W. David Pierce
University of Alberta
Carl D. Cheney
Utah State University

Behavior Analysis and Learning is an essential textbook covering the basic principles in the field of behavior analysis and learned behaviors. Both active researchers, the authors are disciples of a coherent theory—experimental analysis of behavior—pioneered by B.F. Skinner. Using this theory as a base to explain human behavior, researchers must understand the interactions between an individual and his or her environment.

Expanding on concepts of the past editions, this book:
* is an advanced introductory text on operant conditioning from a very consistent Skinnerian perspective;
* covers a range of principles from basic respondent conditioning through applied behavior analysis into cultural design;
* treats the topic from a consistent world view of selectionism;
* elaborates on Darwinian components and biological connections with behavior; and,
* expands most chapters with revised references and additional citations.

The material presented in this book provides the reader with the best available foundation in behavior science. The discovery of functional relations between the organism and the environment constitute the objective foundation for this book. These functional relationships are described, and their application in accounting for old behavior and generating new behavior is illustrated. As such, this book is a valuable resource for advanced undergraduate and graduate students in psychology or other behavior-based disciplines.

Contents: Foreword. Preface. A Science of Behavior: Perspective, History, and Assumptions. The Experimental Analysis of Behavior. Reflexive Behavior and Respondent Conditioning. Reinforcement and Extinction of Operant Behavior. Schedules of Reinforcement. Aversive Control of Behavior. Operant-Respondent Interrelationships and the Biological Context of Conditioning. Stimulus Control. Choice and Preference. Conditioned Reinforcement. Correspondent Relations: Imitation and Rule-Governed Behavior. Verbal Behavior. Applied Behavior Analysis. Three Levels of Selection: Biology, Behavior, and Culture.
0-8058-4489-9 [cloth] / 2004 / 528pp. / $79.95
Prices are subject to change without notice.

Lawrence Erlbaum Associates, Inc.
10 Industrial Ave., Mahwah, NJ 07430–2262
201–258–2200; 1–800–926–6579; fax 201–760–3735
orders@erlbaum.com; www.erlbaum.com

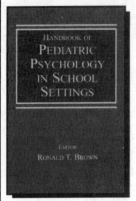